Gastroenterologic Issues in the Obese Patient

Guest Editor

DAVID A. JOHNSON, MD

GASTROENTEROLOGY CLINICS OF NORTH AMERICA

www.gastro.theclinics.com

March 2010 • Volume 39 • Number 1

SAUNDERS an imprint of ELSEVIER, Inc.

W.B. SAUNDERS COMPANY

A Division of Elsevier Inc.

Elsevier Inc. • 1600 John F. Kennedy Blvd., Suite 1800 • Philadelphia, Pennsylvania 19103-2899

http://www.theclinics.com

GASTROENTEROLOGY CLINICS OF NORTH AMERICA Volume 39, Number 1
March 2010 ISSN 0889-8553, ISBN-13: 978-1-4377-1910-9

Editor: Kerry Holland
Developmental Editor: Donald Mumford

Gastroenterology Clinics of North America (ISSN 0889-8553) is published quarterly by Elsevier Inc., 360 Park Avenue South, New York, NY 10010-1710. Months of issue are March, June, September, and December. Business and Editorial Offices: 1600 John F. Kennedy Blvd., Suite 1800, Philadelphia, PA 19103-2899. Customer Service Office: 6277 Sea Harbor Drive, Orlando, FL 32887-4800. Periodicals postage paid at New York, NY and additional mailing offices. Subscription prices are $264.00 per year (US individuals), $135.00 per year (US students), $416.00 per year (US institutions), $290.00 per year (Canadian individuals), $507.00 per year (Canadian institutions), $366.00 per year (international individuals), $186.00 per year (international students), and $507.00 per year (international institutions). Foreign air speed delivery is included in all *Clinics* subscription prices. All prices are subject to change without notice. **POSTMASTER**: Send address changes to *Gastroenterology Clinics of North America*, Elsevier Health Sciences Division, Subscription Customer Service, 3251 Riverport Lane, Maryland Heights, MO 63043. Telephone: 1-800-654-2452 (U.S. and Canada); 314-447-8871 (outside U.S. and Canada). Fax: 314-447-8029. E-mail: journalscustomerservice-usa@elsevier.com (for print support); journalsonlinesupport-usa@elsevier.com (for online support).

Reprints. For copies of 100 or more, of articles in this publication, please contact the Commercial Reprints Department, Elsevier Inc., 360 Part Avenue South, New York, New York 10010-1710. Tel. (212) 633-3813, Fax: (212) 462-1935, E-mail: reprints@elsevier.com.

Gastroenterology Clinics of North America is also published in Italian by Il Pensiero Scientifico Editore, Rome, Italy; and in Portuguese by Interlivros Edicoes Ltda., Rua Commandante Coelho 1085, 21250 Cordovil, Rio de Janeiro, Brazil.

Gastroenterology Clinics of North America is covered in *MEDLINE/PubMed (Index Medicus)*, *Excerpta Medica*, *Current Contents/Clinical Medicine*, *Science Citation Index*, *ISI/BIOMED*, and *BIOSIS*.

Printed and bound by CPI Group (UK) Ltd, Croydon, CR0 4YY

Transferred to Digital Print 2011

Contributors

GUEST EDITOR

DAVID A. JOHNSON, MD, FACG, FASGE
Professor of Medicine, Chief of Gastroenterology, Eastern Virginia Medical School, Norfolk, Virginia

AUTHORS

GIRISH ANAND, MD
Division of Gastroenterology, Albert Einstein Medical Center, Philadelphia, Pennsylvania

CAROL A. BURKE, MD, FACG, FACP
Department of Gastroenterology and Hepatology, Director, Center for Colon Polyp and Cancer Prevention, Digestive Disease Institute, Cleveland Clinic, Cleveland, Ohio

PETER F. CROOKES, MD
Department of Surgery, Keck School of Medicine, University of Southern California, Los Angeles, California

ANNA MAE DIEHL, MD
Professor of Medicine and Chief, Division of Gastroenterology, Duke University, Durham, North Carolina

HASHEM B. EL-SERAG, MD, MPH
Section of Health Services Research, Baylor College of Medicine; Section of Gastroenterology, Baylor College of Medicine; Michael E. DeBakey VA Medical Center, Houston, Texas

GUY D. ESLICK, PhD, MMedSc (Clin Epi), MMedStat
School of Public Health, The University of Sydney, Sydney, New South Wales, Australia; Program in Molecular and Genetic Epidemiology, Department of Epidemiology, Harvard School of Public Health, Boston, Massachusetts

M. BRIAN FENNERTY, MD
Professor of Medicine, Division of Gastroenterology, Oregon Health and Science University, Portland, Oregon

FREDERICK C. FINELLI, MD, JD
Vice President, Performance Improvement and Safety; Department of Surgery, Washington Hospital Center, Washington, DC

MARK A. FONTANA, MD, FACS
Clinical Director, Sentara Metabolic and Weight Loss Surgery Center; Assistant Professor of Surgery, Eastern Virginia Medical School, Norfolk, Virginia

AMY E. FOXX-ORENSTEIN, DO, FACG, FACP
Associate Professor of Medicine, Division of Gastroenterology and Hepatology, Mayo Clinic College of Medicine, Rochester, Minnesota

PAUL FRANK
Department of Surgery, Keck School of Medicine, University of Southern California, Los Angeles, California

DAVID GREENWALD, MD
Fellowship Director in Gastroenterology, Division of Gastroenterology, Montefiore Medical Center; Associate Professor of Clinical Medicine, Albert Einstein College of Medicine, Bronx, New York

LEE M. KAPLAN, MD, PhD
MGH Weight Center and Gastrointestinal Unit, Massachusetts General Hospital and Harvard Medical School, Boston, Massachusetts

PHILIP O. KATZ, MD
Chairman, Division of Gastroenterology, Albert Einstein Medical Center; Clinical Professor of Medicine, Thomas Jefferson University, Philadelphia, Pennsylvania

TIMOTHY R. KOCH, MD, FACG
Professor of Medicine (Gastroenterology), Georgetown University School of Medicine; Department of Surgery, Washington Hospital Center, Washington, DC

TERCIO L. LOPES, MD, MSPH
Division of Gastroenterology and Hepatology, Mayo Clinic College of Medicine, Rochester, Minnesota

DANG M. NGUYEN, MD
Section of Gastroenterology and Hepatology, Baylor College of Medicine; Michael E. DeBakey VA Medical Center, Houston, Texas

MITCHAL A. SCHREINER, MD, MPH
Division of Gastroenterology, Oregon Health and Science University, Portland, Oregon

C. MEL WILCOX, MD, MSPH
Division of Gastroenterology and Hepatology, The University of Alabama at Birmingham, Birmingham, Alabama

STEPHEN D. WOHLGEMUTH, MD, FACS
Program Director, Sentara Metabolic and Weight Loss Surgery Center; Assistant Professor of Surgery, Eastern Virginia Medical School, Norfolk, Virginia

Contents

also common. Obesity and GERD are clearly related, both from a prevalence and causality association. GERD symptoms increase in severity when people gain weight. Obese patients tend to have more severe erosive esophagitis and obesity is a risk factor for the development of Barrett's esophagus and adenocarcinoma of the esophagus. Patients report improvement in GERD when they lose weight and there are several reports suggesting a decrease in GERD symptoms after bariatric surgery. At present, there is little evidence that obesity has any effect on the efficacy of antisecretory therapy, with conflicting data on surgical outcomes. This review attempts to put in perspective the relationship of these two common entities.

Obesity is a risk factor for colorectal cancer and adenomatous polyps. The increased prevalence of neoplasia coupled with the observation that obesity may be associated with a suboptimal bowel preparation may diminish the adequate detection of adenomas for obese who undergo colonoscopy. The colonic complications of obesity are reviewed in this article.

Obesity is associated with a spectrum of chronic liver disease. Because obesity increases the risk for advanced forms of liver disease (ie, cirrhosis and liver cancer), the obesity epidemic is emerging as a major factor underlying the burden of liver disease in the United States and many other countries. This article reviews mechanisms that mediate the pathogenesis of obesity-related liver disease, summarizes clinical evidence that demonstrates obesity-related liver disease can be life-threatening, and discusses whether or not treatments for obesity or related comorbidities impact liver disease outcomes.

This article examines the transitions in pharmacological therapy for obesity. It reviews the current options approved by the Food and Drug Administration and several drugs approved for other indications that can be used to treat obesity as well. Because weight regulation is complex and redundant systems protect against perceived starvation, optimal treatment of obesity in individual patients will likely require different combinations of behavioral, nutritional, pharmacologic, endoscopic, and surgical therapies.

Obesity is a major health problem throughout the world. Bariatric surgery is frequently considered among the treatment options for the severely overweight, and surgically induced weight loss has become the best treatment for many morbidly obese people. A preoperative assessment to evaluate the suitability of a patient for a given operation and to clarify factors that may affect the outcome of a planned procedure should be carried out before the surgery. Preoperative evaluation of the gastrointestinal tract by a gastroenterologist before bariatric surgery yields important information that can lead to changes in planned treatments. This article discusses the factors that a gastroenterologist should assess before the surgery.

Mitchal A. Schreiner and M. Brian Fennerty

Obese patients present many unique challenges to the endoscopist. Special consideration should be given to these patients, and endoscopists need to be aware of the additional challenges that may be present while performing endoscopic procedures on obese patients. This article reviews the special risks that obese patients face while undergoing endoscopy, endoscopic management of patients postbariatric surgery, and future role of endoscopy in the management of obese patients.

Tercio L. Lopes and C. Mel Wilcox

Bariatric surgery has been increasingly performed in response to the obesity pandemic. During the last decade, Roux-en-Y gastric bypass (RYGB) has become the preferred surgical approach. It is also commonly performed after pylorus preserving pancreaticoduodenectomy and other biliary tract surgeries. This article discusses the different options available for endoscopists who are faced with the need to perform endoscopic retrograde cholangiopancreatography in patients after Roux-en-Y reconstruction, with special emphasis on those after RYGB.

Timothy R. Koch and Frederick C. Finelli

Bariatric surgery has become an increasingly important method for management of medically complicated obesity. In patients who have undergone bariatric surgery, up to 87% with type 2 diabetes mellitus develop improvement or resolution of their disease postoperatively. Bariatric surgery can reduce the number of absorbed calories through performance of either a restrictive or a malabsorptive procedure. Patients who have undergone bariatric surgery require indefinite, regular follow-up care by physicians who need to follow laboratory parameters of macronutrient as well as micronutrient malnutrition. Physicians who care for patients after bariatric surgery need to be familiar with common postoperative syndromes that result from specific nutrient deficiencies.

The disease of obesity has continued to increase in the United States. Obesity is defined as a body mass index (BMI) greater than 30 kg/m². In 1991, the National Institute of Health Consensus Panel on Gastric Surgery for Severe Obesity defined the population who would most likely benefit from bariatric surgery. These same criteria continue to be used today to determine which patients should undergo metabolic and weight loss surgery. These recommendations include patients who have a BMI greater than 35 kg/m² with significant comorbid conditions such as diabetes, hypertension, or obstructive sleep apnea; and patients who have a BMI greater than 40 kg/m² with or without any significant comorbid conditions because they have a significant increased risk for developing these conditions.

Follow-up of the large numbers of patients undergoing bariatric surgery poses problems for surgical programs and for internists who care for morbidly obese patients. Early surgical follow up is concentrated on the perioperative period to ensure healing and care for any surgical complications. It is especially important to treat persistent vomiting to avoid thiamine deficiency. Subsequently, monitoring weight loss and resolution of comorbidities assumes more importance. Identification and management of nutritional deficiencies and other unwanted consequences of surgery may become the responsibility of internists if the patient no longer attends the office of the operating surgeon. The long-term goal is to avoid weight regain and deficiencies, especially of protein, iron and vitamin B12, and calcium and vitamin D. Abdominal pain and gastrointestinal dysfunction should be investigated promptly to exclude or confirm such conditions as small bowel obstruction or gallstones. Good communication between bariatric surgeons and internal medicine specialists is essential for early and accurate identification of problems arising from bariatric surgery.

THE CLINICS ARE NOW AVAILABLE ONLINE!

Access your subscription at:
www.theclinics.com

Preface

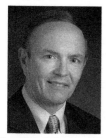

David A. Johnson, MD
Guest Editor

Obesity has emerged as a major global health problem with disease prevalence reaching epidemic proportions. In the United States alone, obesity is responsible for more than 300,000 deaths per year. Additionally, the direct and indirect related costs for care of obesity-related disease exceed $100 billion per year. Obesity has a particular relevance to gastroenterologists given the wide spectrum of causally related disease implications specific to this specialty. It is increasingly apparent that obesity has significant implications for gastrointestinal diseases and increased risks of serious consequences, including cancer. Gastroenterologists are increasingly involved in the care of obese and overweight patients. This involvement includes assessing for appropriate screening for neoplasia, as well as conducting evaluations or interventions pre- or postoperatively.

In the first article, Drs Dang Nguyen and Hashem El-Serag define the scope of the obesity problem. Over the last 3 decades, overindulgence and obesity have been transformed from a relatively minor public health issue affecting affluent societies to a current global epidemic with major public health implications. This article puts into perspective the epidemiologic implications, in particular for gastrointestinal-related diseases.

In the next two articles, the focus is on gastrointestinal symptoms in obese patients. The role of gastrointestinal symptoms in overweight and obese individuals has only barely been explored, which is surprising given that the gastrointestinal tract is responsible for the mechanical and chemical breakdown of food for absorption by the body. Dr Guy Eslick puts into perspective the prevalence of particular gastrointestinal symptoms correlated with increased body weight. Dr Amy Foxx-Orenstein follows with an excellent summary of the physiologic explanations for this correlation of increased gastrointestinal symptoms as a function of body habitus.

Gastroesophageal reflux disease is an extremely prevalent disease and there is increasing evidence to support a causal relationship with obesity for both disease prevalence as well as complications. Drs Girish Anand and Phil Katz detail the most recent evidence for mechanistic explanations for causality and highlight the increased

Gastroenterol Clin N Am 39 (2010) xi–xiii
doi:10.1016/j.gtc.2009.12.013
0889-8553/10/$ – see front matter © 2010 Elsevier Inc. All rights reserved.

severity and complications of gastroesophageal reflux disease in this specific patient population.

While the most studied effect of obesity is on its association with colorectal neoplasia, lesser known effects include a heightened risk of complications of diverticulosis, a heightened risk inadequate bowel preparation, and a poorer, postoperative outcome after colon surgery. Dr Carol Burke provides a comprehensive update on the effects of obesity on colonic diseases and complications. The review highlights the emerging data showing that adverse effects of obesity on the colon promote carcinogenesis and impair wound healing. This has implications for appropriate screening as well as surgical management of the obese patient.

Nonalcoholic fatty liver disease is a very common clinical condition evident as a complication of obesity. The spectrum of liver histologic abnormalities ranges from simple steatosis to steatohepatitis, advanced fibrosis, and cirrhosis. Dr Anna Mae Diehl provides an outstanding overview of the comorbid diseases associated with obesity-related liver disease and then reviews the clinical features, management strategies, and prognosis for this extremely prevalent problem.

The medical management for obesity is a key area of interest. Pharmacologic therapy for obesity is clearly in a state of transition. Historically, there have been few effective agents, and many have been withdrawn because of unacceptable side effects. Given the widespread prevalence of obesity, there is intense interest in a nonsurgical option for treatment. Dr Lee Kaplan details the past, present, and future medications for the medical therapy option. His article focuses on key areas of interest to providers taking care of patients who are on these agents and highlights potential side effects and complications related to these medications.

Gastroenterologists are becoming increasingly involved in both the preoperative and postoperative care of bariatric patients. Accordingly, it is key for gastroenterologists (and those dealing with gastrointestinal-related issues) to understand the full spectrum of assessment and management. This ranges from both the preoperative evaluation for gastrointestinal-related disease to management of a wide array of endoscopic interventions and metabolic complications postoperatively. Dr David Greenwald begins the discussion with the gastrointestinal role in the preoperative assessment of bariatric patients. Drs Mitch Schreiner and Brian Fennerty focus in particular on the standard endoscopic assessment and management both pre- and postoperatively. Drs Tercio Lopes and Mel Wilcox then address the approach to the postoperative bariatric patient with pancreaticobiliary disease and provide insight and technical expertise dealing with the altered anatomy. Dr Tim Koch then provides an excellent overview on the wide array of metabolic complications for the postoperative bariatric patient. His review highlights the macro- and micronutrient potential deficiencies and he provides a comprehensive approach to both the short- and long-term management to treat or potentially avoid these complications.

Bariatric surgery is the most definitive treatment for obesity. As bariatric surgery has gained widespread acceptance, evidence continues to grow that it is the only treatment currently available that demonstrates significant cure rates for such diseases as diabetes, hypertension, and heart failure, as well as the myriad of other comorbid conditions associated with obesity. In 2008, at least 220,000 obesity surgeries were done in the United States, with gastric bypass being the "most popular method." Drs Mark Fontana and Steve Wohlgemuth review the weight-loss surgery options. The emphasis is on the common operations performed currently, but they also discuss operations no longer performed. Knowledge of the anatomic changes is key to understanding and optimizing management strategies of the short- and long-term postoperative complications. Drs Paul Frank and Peter Crookes provide the surgeon's perspective for the short- and long-term follow up of the postbariatric surgery patient. They emphasize that, although early surgical follow up is concentrated on the perioperative period to ensure healing and care for any surgical complications, the key element of ultimate "surgical success" is the long-term programmatic follow up for these patients. These authors provide recommendations drawing from their extensive experience with the comprehensive program used at their institution.

Recognizably from this edition of *Gastroenterology Clinics of North America*, obesity is a major risk factor for a range of serious medical conditions, including a wide spectrum of gastrointestinal-related disorders and complications. The complex metabolic activity of adipose tissue results in the production of proinflammatory cytokines and neurohumoral and immune-mediated mechanisms, leading to a host of systemic effects, which include a broad array of gastrointestinal symptoms and diseases.

So where do we go from here? All medical practitioners, including gastroenterologists and bariatric surgeons, must remain aggressive about addressing and treating obesity in their patients. This monograph will, it is hoped, be a key step in advancing the knowledge base of those who care for obese patients. Furthermore, it is the collective intent of the authors that this will also highlight the absolute need for a comprehensive, well-integrated multidisciplinary and *lifelong* approach to these patients.

David A. Johnson, MD
Department of Gastroenterology
885 Kempsville Road, Suite 114
Norfolk, VA 23505, USA

E-mail address:
dajevms@aol.com

The Epidemiology of Obesity

Dang M. Nguyen, MD[a,b], Hashem B. El-Serag, MD, MPH[a,b,c],*

KEYWORDS

- Obesity • Epidemiology of obesity
- Complications of obesity • Genetic basis

Obesity has received considerable attention as a major health hazard. This article describes some of the epidemiologic features of obesity, including global prevalence, secular trends, risk factors, and burden of illness related to obesity. Special emphasis is placed on obesity trends in the United States.

DEFINITIONS FOR OVERWEIGHT AND OBESITY

The techniques that measure body composition include densitometry, single-cut imaging of the abdomen using computed tomography (CT) scan or magnetic resonance imaging (MRI), and dual-energy X-ray absorptiometry, but these methods are used mostly for research purposes. Body mass index (BMI), which is calculated as the weight in kilograms divided by the height in meters squared (kg/m^2), is the most widely used measure of obesity because of its low cost and simplicity. The World Health Organization (WHO) and the National Institutes of Health[1,2] define a person to be overweight when he or she has a BMI between 25.0 and 29.9 kg/m^2; and a person to be obese when he or she has a BMI greater than 30.0 kg/m^2. In the United States, the criteria for categorizing children as overweight are based on the 2000 US Centers for Disease Control and Prevention's (CDC) BMI-for-age growth charts. According to these charts a person is considered to be overweight when he or she has a BMI at or above the age-specific 95% BMI percentile. At risk for overweight is a condition when the BMI falls between the 85th and 95th percentiles of the BMI-for-age growth charts.[3]

This research was partially supported by the grant R01 titled "Obesity, H pylori, and risk of Barrett esophagus," and the grant K24 titled "Epidemiology and outcomes of digestive and liver diseases." It was also partly supported by the Houston VA HSR&D Center of Excellence (HFP90-020).

a Section of Gastroenterology and Hepatology, Baylor College of Medicine, Houston, TX, USA
b Michael E. DeBakey VA Medical Center, 2002 Holcombe Boulevard (MS 152), Houston, TX 77030, USA
c Section of Health Services Research, Baylor College of Medicine, Houston, TX, USA
* Corresponding author. Michael E. DeBakey VA Medical Center, 2002 Holcombe Boulevard (MS 152), Houston, TX 77030.
E-mail address: hasheme@bcm.tmc.edu

However, increasing evidence suggests that abdominal obesity, rather than total body fat, is also a useful, independent predictor of several cardiovascular-related outcomes and cancer-related outcomes.[2] Some of the commonly used measures of abdominal obesity are waist circumference, hip circumference, and waist-to-hip ratio.

OBESITY TRENDS IN ADULTS AND CHILDREN
Obesity Trends in Adults in the United States

A few important sources of epidemiologic data on obesity in the United States are discussed in this article.

The Behavioral Risk Factor Surveillance System (BRFSS) is a state-based cross-sectional random telephone survey of the population of United States of age greater than or equal to 18 years. At the time of the survey, BMI was calculated from self-reported weight and height.[3] The 2008 BRFSS data showed considerable differences in the prevalence of obesity across states. Five states (Alabama, Mississippi, Oklahoma, Tennessee, and West Virginia) had a prevalence of obesity equal to or greater than 30%, and 32 states had a prevalence of obesity equal to or greater than 25%. For comparison, in 1990, no state had a prevalence of obesity greater than 15%; 10 states had a prevalence of obesity less than 10%, and the rest had an obesity prevalence of 10% to 15%.[3]

The National Health and Nutrition Examination Survey (NHANES) is another cross-sectional, nationally representative series of surveys conducted by the National Center for Health Statistics of the US CDC. All surveys included a standardized physical examination, with the measurement of weight and height using standardized protocols that were conducted in a mobile examination center.[4,5] According to NHANES data for the 2003 to 2004 period, 66.2% of the adults in the United States who were between the age of 20 and 74 years were either overweight or obese, 33.4% were overweight, and 32.9% were obese. Recent data from NHANES show no significant changes in the prevalence of obesity for either men or women between 2003 to 2004 and 2005 to 2006 (**Figs. 1 and 2**).[6,7] This possible stabilization in the obesity trends may be an early sign of a plateau in the obesity epidemic. The prevalence of obesity was relatively low and stable between 1960 and 1980, but more than doubled from 15% in 1980 to 34% in 2006.[6,7]

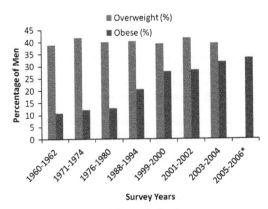

Fig. 1. Prevalence and trends of overweight and obesity among men aged 20 to 74 years in the United States from 1960 to 2006. *Included all people older than 20 years; only data in obese category are available.

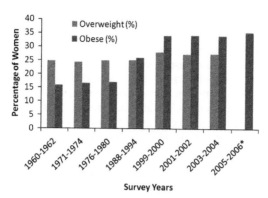

Fig. 2. Prevalence and trends of overweight and obesity among women aged 20 to 74 years in the United States from 1960 to 2006. *Included all people older than 20 years; only data in obese category are available.

Data from NHANES show large ethnic differences in the prevalence of obesity, but do not include an adequate number of minorities other than African Americans and Mexican Americans. Based on the data from NHANES for the period 2003 to 2004, African Americans had the highest prevalence of obesity at 45% for men and women between the age of 20 and 74 years; the obesity prevalence was 30.6% for Caucasians and 36.8% for Mexican Americans.[7] The data from NHANES for the period 2005 to 2006 show large differences in obesity prevalence among women belonging to different ethnic groups and between the age of 40 and 59 years, but no significant differences among men belonging to the same ethnic groups. Approximately 53% of African-American women and 51% of Mexican-American women were obese, compared with 39% of Caucasian women.[6]

Overweight Trends in Children in the United States

National estimates of overweight or obesity in children based on the NHANES data show that during the period 2003 to 2006, 31.9% of children aged 2 to 19 years had a BMI at or above the 85th percentile of the 2000 CDC BMI-for-age growth charts, and 16.3% had a BMI at or above the 95th percentile of that chart. Recent data from NHANES show no significant changes in the prevalence of obesity for children aged 2 to 19 years between 2003 to 2004 and 2005 to 2006.[8] The overweight prevalence changed dramatically between 1980 and 2006 for children aged 2 to 19 years, increasing from 5.5% in 1980 to 16.3% in 2006.

Global Trends of Obesity

The current epidemic of obesity has been reported in several but not all regions globally. The highest rate of obesity has been reported in the Pacific Islands and the lowest rates have been seen in Asia. The rates in Europe and North America are generally high, whereas the rates in Africa and Middle Eastern countries are variable.[9] The prevalence of obesity around the world is monitored by the WHO through the Global Database on BMI. The survey data included in the database are identified from the literature or from a wide network of collaborators. However, high-quality data from systematic nationally representative samples is sparse. As of November 2004, the database has compiled data covering approximately 86% of the adult population worldwide.[1] The WHO estimates showed that in 2005, approximately 1.6 billion people worldwide were overweight and that at least 400 million adults were obese. The WHO further projects that by 2015, approximately 2.3 billion adults will be overweight and that at least 700 million will be obese. According to the data from the Global Database on BMI, there are wide variations in the prevalence of obesity throughout the world, ranging from India, where 1% or less of the population is obese, to the Pacific Islands, where the prevalence of obesity can reach up to 80% in some regions.[1]

The change in adult obesity prevalence over time was calculated for 28 countries that have 2 or more nationally representative surveys recorded in the Global Database on BMI. Overall, most countries were found to have rising trends of obesity. Only 2 (Denmark and Saudi Arabia) of the 28 countries showed a falling trend in the prevalence of obesity in men, and 5 (Denmark, Ireland, Saudi Arabia, Finland, and Spain) of the 28 countries showed a falling trend in the prevalence of obesity in women.[10]

POSSIBLE CAUSES OF THE OBESITY EPIDEMIC

Obesity is caused by a complex interaction of the environment, the genetic predisposition, and human behavior.

Environmental factors are likely to be major contributors to the obesity epidemic. It is certain that obesity develops when there is a positive imbalance between energy intake and energy expenditure, but the relative contribution of these factors is poorly understood. Evidence supports the contribution of excess energy intake and decreased energy expenditure in the obesity epidemic.[11-13] Kant and Graubard[11] used dietary data from 4 consecutive NHANES studies consisting of 39,094 adults in the United States to show that the temporal trends in the increase of the quantity and energy density of foods consumed by adults parallel the increasing prevalence of obesity of the population in the United States. Data from the Central Statistical Office show that rising car ownership and increasing television viewing, which are proxy measures of physical inactivity, closely parallel the rising trends in obesity in England.[12] Using data from NHANES, Dietz and Gortmaker[13] showed that the prevalence of obesity increased by 2% for each additional hour of television viewed. There is also evidence that the relative availability and price of different food products affect food consumption,[14] and that the built environment, such as quality of local parks, affects the level of physical activities in a community.[15] These findings not only emphasize the impact of environmental factors on the obesity epidemic but also indicate that policies affecting the availability of high caloric density food, the cost of fruits and vegetables, and the built environment may contribute to the obesity epidemic.

In addition to environmental factors, there is genetic predisposition to obesity. It is known that single gene mutations are responsible for rare forms of monogenic obesity (leptin [LEP], leptin receptor [LEPR], melanocortin-4 receptor [MC4R], and pro-opiomelanocortin [POMC]).[16] However, there is growing evidence that common genetic variants or single nucleotide polymorphisms (SNPs) may play an important role in the obesity epidemic. These SNPs have modest effects on an individual's susceptibility to common forms of obesity, but because of their high frequency, they can have a large contribution to obesity on the population level.[17] Frayling and colleagues[18] were the first to use a genome-wide (GWA) study to identify an SNP located in the fat mass and obesity gene (FTO) an obesity susceptibility gene. The finding that the FTO gene variant is a risk factor for common obesity has now been replicated in multiples studies.[19-21] FTO has been identified in a GWA study to be associated with an increased risk of type 2 diabetes mediated through an effect on the BMI. In a GWA study of 38,759 patients, Frayling and colleagues[18] found that a person who is homozygous for the risk allele (rs9939609 A allele) of FTO had a 1.67-fold increased odds of obesity when compared with those who do not have the risk allele.

There is growing recognition that social networks may have an important role in the obesity epidemic. Christakis and Fowler[22] explored the hypothesis that obesity may spread through social networks by evaluating an interconnected social network of more than 12,000 people from the Framingham Heart Study to examine the effects of weight gain among friends, siblings, and spouses. These investigators found that a person's risk of becoming obese increased by 57% if a friend became obese. The association was smaller among siblings and spouses: the risk of becoming obese increased by 40% and 37% if a person had a sibling or spouse who became obese, respectively.[22] By exploring the role of social networks and obesity, this study showed that the obesity epidemic is affected by the complex interaction between the environment, genetic factors, and human behavior (eg, passive permission).

BURDEN OF ILLNESS ASSOCIATED WITH OBESITY

Obesity is associated with an increased risk of death. Adams and colleagues[23] estimated the risk of death in a prospective cohort of more than 500,000 men and women from the United States after 10 years of follow-up, and reported that among patients who had never smoked, the risk of death is increased by 20% to 40% in overweight patients and by two- to threefold in obese compared with normal-weight patients.

Obesity is also associated with increased risk for numerous chronic diseases, including diabetes, hypertension, heart disease, and stroke.[24] Furthermore, obesity is linked to several digestive diseases, including gastroesophageal reflux disease and its complications (eg, erosive esophagitis, Barrett esophagus, and esophageal adenocarcinoma), colorectal polyps and cancer, and liver disease (eg, nonalcoholic fatty liver disease, cirrhosis, and hepatocellular carcinoma).[25]

Because of the increased risk of death and the increased risk of costly chronic diseases associated with obesity, the obesity epidemic places a large financial burden on the economy. The US Department of Health and Human Services has estimated the total economic cost of overweight and obesity in the United States to be close to $117 billion using data from 1995, updated to 2001 dollars.[26] However, because the prevalence of overweight and obesity have increased since 1995, the costs today are likely to be considerably higher than previous estimates. Trogdon and colleagues,[27] based on data from a systematic review, estimated that the total indirect cost in the United States for 1999 was $65.67 billion. A recent study by Finkelstein and colleagues[28] projected that the annual medical spending because of overweight and obesity approached $92.6 billion in 2002, which constitutes about 9% of health expenditure in the United States.[26]

SUMMARY AND CONCLUSIONS

The prevalence of obesity in the United States has increased dramatically since 1980 in both adults and children. However, there is evidence of a possible recent stabilization from data that compares obesity in the 2003 to 2004 period with that in the 2005 to 2006 period for children and adults in the United States The epidemic of obesity is not limited to the United States but has been documented in several regions worldwide, with the prevalence of obesity rising in most countries. Obesity is affected by a complex interaction between the environment, genetic predisposition, and human behavior; it is associated with an increased risk of numerous chronic diseases, from diabetes and cancers to many digestive diseases. In addition, the obesity epidemic exerts a heavy toll on the economy with its massive health care costs. The problem of overweight and obesity has therefore emerged as one of the most pressing global issues to be faced during the next several decades, and it hence demands attention from the health care community, researchers, and policy makers. The implications for gastrointestinal health care providers are readily apparent and will be addressed in the text of this entire issue of *Gastroenterology Clinics*.

REFERENCES

1. World Health Organization. Obesity 2008. Available at: http://www.who.int/topics/obesity/en/. Accessed October 22, 2009.
2. Kumanyika SK, Obarzanek E, Stettler N, et al. Population-based prevention of obesity: the need for comprehensive promotion of healthful eating, physical activity, and energy balance: a scientific statement from American Heart Association Council on Epidemiology and Prevention, Interdisciplinary Committee for Prevention (formerly the expert panel on population and prevention science). Circulation 2008;118(4):428–64.
3. US Centers for Disease control and Prevention. Overweight and obesity 2008. Available at: http://www.cdc.gov/nccdphp/dnpa/obesity/trend/maps/index.htm. Accessed October 22, 2009.
4. Ogden CL, Flegal KM, Carroll MD, et al. Prevalence and trends in overweight among US children and adolescents, 1999–2000. JAMA 2002;288(14):1728–32.
5. Flegal KM, Carroll MD, Ogden CL, et al. Prevalence and trends in obesity among US adults, 1999–2000. JAMA 2002;288(14):1723–7.
6. Ogden CL, Carroll MD, McDowell MA, et al. Obesity among adults in the United States—no change since 2003-2004. NCHS data brief no 1 National Center for Health Statistics 2007.
7. Ogden CL, Yanovski SZ, Carroll MD, et al. The epidemiology of obesity. Gastroenterology 2007;132(6):2087–102.
8. Ogden CL, Carroll MD, Flegal KM. High body mass index for age among US children and adolescents, 2003–2006. JAMA 2008;299(20):2401–5.
9. Prentice AM. The emerging epidemic of obesity in developing countries. Int J Epidemiol 2006;35(1):93–9.
10. Nishida C, Mucavele P. Monitoring the rapidly emerging public health problem of overweight and obesity: the WHO Global Database on body mass index. SCN News 2005;29:5–12.
11. Kant AK, Graubard BI. Secular trends in patterns of self-reported food consumption of adult Americans: NHANES 1971–1975 to NHANES 1999–2002. Am J Clin Nutr 2006;84(5):1215–23.
12. Prentice AM, Jebb SA. Obesity in Britain: gluttony or sloth? BMJ 1995;311(7002):437–9.
13. Dietz WH Jr, Gortmaker SL. Do we fatten our children at the television set? Obesity and television viewing in children and adolescents. Pediatrics 1985;75(5):807–12.
14. Holsten JE. Obesity and the community food environment: a systematic review. Public Health Nutr 2008;12:1–9.
15. Kipke MD, Iverson E, Moore D, et al. Food and park environments: neighborhood-level risks for childhood obesity in east Los Angeles. J Adolesc Health 2007;40(4):325–33.
16. Andreasen CH, Andersen G. Gene-environment interactions and obesity—further aspects of genomewide association studies. Nutrition 2009;25(10):998–1003.

17. Tiret L, Poirier O, Nicaud V, et al. Heterogeneity of linkage disequilibrium in human genes has implications for association studies of common diseases. Hum Mol Genet 2002;11(4):419–29.
18. Frayling TM, Timpson NJ, Weedon MN, et al. A common variant in the FTO gene is associated with body mass index and predisposes to childhood and adult obesity. Science 2007;316(5826):889–94.
19. Hunt SC, Stone S, Xin Y, et al. Association of the FTO gene with BMI. Obesity (Silver Spring) 2008;16(4):902–4.
20. Haupt A, Thamer C, Machann J, et al. Impact of variation in the FTO gene on whole body fat distribution, ectopic fat, and weight loss. Obesity (Silver Spring) 2008;16(8):1969–72.
21. Andreasen CH, Stender-Petersen KL, Mogensen MS, et al. Low physical activity accentuates the effect of the FTO rs9939609 polymorphism on body fat accumulation. Diabetes 2008;57(1):95–101.
22. Christakis NA, Fowler JH. The spread of obesity in a large social network over 32 years. N Engl J Med 2007;357(4):370–9.
23. Adams KF, Schatzkin A, Harris TB, et al. Overweight, obesity, and mortality in a large prospective cohort of persons 50 to 71 years old. N Engl J Med 2006; 355(8):763–78.
24. Field AE, Coakley EH, Must A, et al. Impact of overweight on the risk of developing common chronic diseases during a 10-year period. Arch Intern Med 2001;161(13):1581–6.
25. American College of Gastroenterology. Obesity and digestive disorders a physician reference 2008. Available at: http://www.acg.gi.org/obesity/pdfs/ACG_Obesity_Physician_Reference.pdf. Accessed November 9, 2008.
26. NIDDK Weight Control Information Network. Statistics related to overweight and obesity Economic costs related to overweight and obesity 2008. Available at: http://win.niddk.nih.gov/statist. Accessed November 9, 2008.
27. Trogdon JG, Finkelstein EA, Hylands T, et al. Indirect costs of obesity: a review of the current literature. Obes Rev 2008;9(5):489–500.
28. Finkelstein EA, Fiebelkorn IC, Wang G. State-level estimates of annual medical expenditures attributable to obesity. Obes Res 2004;12(1):18–24.

Prevalence and Epidemiology of Gastrointestinal Symptoms Among Normal Weight, Overweight, Obese and Extremely Obese Individuals

Guy D. Eslick, PhD, MMedSc (Clin Epi), MMedStat[a,b,*]

KEYWORDS

- Obesity • Epidemiology • Gastrointestinal symptoms
- Ethnicity

The obesity epidemic has brought with it a barrage of comorbid conditions, medical and psychological complications, and complex patients for the physician to interpret.[1–5] Studies on the role of gastrointestinal (GI) symptoms in overweight and obese individuals have been very limited, which is surprising given that the GI tract is responsible for the mechanical and chemical breakdown of food for absorption by the body. The prevalence of those classified as overweight in the United States has not changed much since the 1960s, however, there has been a significant almost threefold increase in the prevalence of obesity that started in 1976 to 1980 and peaked in 1999 to 2000. The largest increase has occurred in the extremely obese category; there has been a sevenfold increase in prevalence in this category between 1960 and 2006 (**Fig. 1**).[6,7] In the middle of this epidemic of increasing body mass index (BMI,

Guy D. Eslick is supported by The International Union Against Cancer (UICC) and the American Cancer Society (ACS) with an International Fellowship for Beginning Investigators (ACSBI).
[a] School of Public Health, The University of Sydney, Sydney, New South Wales, Australia
[b] Program in Molecular and Genetic Epidemiology, Department of Epidemiology, Harvard School of Public Health, 677 Huntington Avenue, Building 2, 2nd Floor, Room 209, Boston, MA 02115, USA
* Program in Molecular and Genetic Epidemiology, Department of Epidemiology, Harvard School of Public Health, 677 Huntington Avenue, Building 2, 2nd Floor, Room 209, Boston, MA 02115.
E-mail address: geslick@hsph.harvard.edu

Gastroenterol Clin N Am 39 (2010) 9–22
doi:10.1016/j.gtc.2009.12.007
0889-8553/10/$ – see front matter. Published by Elsevier Inc.

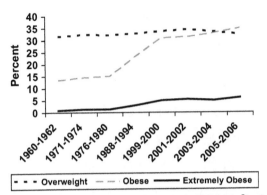

Fig. 1. Age-adjusted prevalence for overweight (BMI 25.0–29.9 kg/m²), obese (BMI 30.0–34.9 kg/m²), and extremely obese (BMI >40.0 kg/m²), among adults in the United States, age 20–74 years (CDC).

calculated as weight in kilograms divided by the square of height in meters) in the United States, the first study assessing the epidemiology of digestive symptoms was conducted at the Johns Hopkins Weight Management Center in 1994. The study aimed to determine the prevalence of GI symptoms among obese and normal weight binge eaters.[8]

It was almost a decade later when a patient-based study of morbidly obese patients undergoing laproscopic Roux-en Y gastric bypass reported substantial increases in GI symptoms compared with normal controls.[9] Following this initial report, there were 3 population-based studies from the United States, New Zealand, and Australia that provided new information about the prevalence of GI symptoms among various BMI categories (normal 18.5–24.9 kg/m², overweight 25.0–29.9 kg/m², obese class I 30.0–34.9 kg/m², obese class II 35.0–39.9 kg/m², and obese class III >40.0 kg/m²).[10–12] Subsequently, there have been an 5 more studies including 2 from Europe,[13,14] 2 from the United States,[15,16] and a recent study from Iran.[17] Moreover, there have been other studies that have provided limited information because of the groups assessed or the variables selected in these studies.[8,18] Despite the global prevalence of obesity, it is evident from the literature that there are few studies assessing the epidemiology of GI symptoms among overweight, obese, or extremely obese individuals either in the community or among patients in the clinical setting.

This review focus only on studies that have aimed to determine the prevalence of multiple GI symptoms in either patient-based samples or in the community (**Table 1**).

GASTROINTESTINAL SYMPTOMS

The studies published so far have assessed 47 GI symptoms (**Box 1**). These consist of upper and lower GI symptoms. The most common symptom assessed in these studies was abdominal pain with 7 out of 9 studies reporting an overall abdominal pain; only 2 studies reported upper and lower abdominal pain as separate symptoms.[10,12] Upper GI symptoms included acid regurgitation, gastroesophageal reflux disease (GERD), dysphagia, vomiting, heartburn, dyspepsia, retching, and nausea; lower GI symptoms included constipation, diarrhea, fecal incontinence, incomplete evacuation, and anal blockage. Some symptoms were commonly reported in 4 or more studies and these included acid regurgitation, bloating, constipation, diarrhea, dysphagia, heartburn, nausea, and vomiting. Although irritable bowel syndrome

Table 1
Characteristics of studies assessing GI symptoms among overweight and obese individuals

Study	Year	Country	Total (n)	Weight Classification	Study Design	Study Sample	GI Symptoms
Foster et al[9]	2003	United States	43	BMI	Cross-sectional	Patient	Abdominal pain, GERD, IBS, reflux, dysphagia
Delgado-Aros et al[10]	2004	United States	1963	BMI	Cross-sectional	Population	Nausea, vomiting, satiety, upper abdominal pain, lower abdominal pain, bloating, diarrhea, constipation
Talley et al[11]	2004	New Zealand	980	BMI	Cohort	Population	Abdominal pain, bloating, heartburn, acid regurgitation, diarrhea, constipation, IBS
Talley et al[12]	2004	Australia	777	Increased BMI	Cross-sectional	Population	Nausea, vomiting, early satiety, upper abdominal pain, lower abdominal pain, bloating, postprandial fullness, hard stools, decreased stools, increased stools, loose watery stools, heartburn, acid regurgitation
Aro et al[13]	2005	Sweden	983	BMI	Cross-sectional	Population	Dysphagia, fullness, retching, acid regurgitation, early satiety, nausea, vomiting, heartburn, central chest pain, burning feeling rising in chest, constipation, diarrhea, incomplete evacuation, pain at defecation, pain relieved at defecation, straining, urgency, flatus, abdominal distention, nightly urge to defecate
van Oijen et al[14]	2006	Netherlands	1023	BMI	Cross-sectional	Patient	Acid regurgitation, heartburn, dyspepsia, GERD, lower abdominal pain
Cremonini et al[15]	2006	United States	637	Weight loss/gain	Cohort	Population	Dyspepsia, GERD, chest pain, dyspepsia dysmotility, dyspepsia pain
Cremonini et al[16]	2009	United States	4096	BMI	Cross-sectional	Population	Abdominal pain, fullness, food staying in stomach, bloating, acid regurgitation, heartburn, nausea, vomiting, dysphagia, anal blockage, diarrhea, constipation, lumpy/hard stools, loose/watery stools, fecal urgency, fecal incontinence
Pourhoseingholi et al[17]	2009	Iran	2790	BMI	Cross-sectional	Population	Abdominal pain, constipation, diarrhea, bloating, heartburn, anal pain, anal bleeding, nausea and vomiting, dysphagia, incontinence

Box 1
GI symptoms reported in studies conducted among obese individuals

- Abdominal distention
- Abdominal pain
- Abdominal pain, upper
- Abdominal pain, lower
- Acid regurgitation
- Anal blockage
- Anal pain
- Anal bleeding
- Bloating
- Burning feeling rising in chest
- Central chest pain
- Chest pain
- Constipation
- Decreased stools
- Diarrhea
- Dysmotility
- Dyspepsia
- Dyspepsia dymotility
- Dyspepsia pain
- Dysphagia
- Early satiety
- Epigastric pain
- Fecal incontinence
- Fecal urgency
- Flatus
- Food staying in stomach
- Frequent stools
- Fullness
- Gastroesophageal reflux disease (GERD)
- Hard stools
- Heartburn
- Incomplete evacuation
- Increased stools
- Irritable bowel syndrome (IBS)
- Loose/watery stools
- Lumpy/hard stools
- Nausea
- Nightly urge to defecate

- Pain at defecation
- Pain relieved at defecation
- Postprandial fullness
- Reflux
- Retching
- Satiety
- Straining
- Urgency
- Vomiting

(IBS) is a syndrome and not a categoric symptom, this was included because the data were available from the studies.

STUDIES EVALUATING GI SYMPTOMS AND OBESITY
Crowell and Colleagues 1994

The aim of this patient-based study was to compare GI symptoms in obese and non-obese binge eaters as defined by DSM-IV.[8] This study was conducted in the United States. There were 119 obese and 77 normal weight women who completed a validated self-report Bowel Symptom Questionnaire (BSQ) and reported GI symptoms in the previous 3-month period. The obese (clinic) patients were significantly younger than the normal weight (community) subjects (45.9 vs 52.0 years, $P<.01$). Multiple GI symptoms were reported more frequently among the obese binge eaters than the normal weight controls ($P<.001$). The prevalence of certain GI symptoms was statistically significant (all $P<.05$) when comparing obese and nonobese groups: flatus (58% vs 39%), constipation (42% vs 23%), diarrhea (35% vs 19%), straining (32% vs 16%), respectively. These were the only symptoms for which prevalence estimates between obese and nonobese groups were reported in this study.

Foster and Colleagues 2003

This patient-based study from the United States compared the prevalence of GI symptoms among 43 (40 female, 3 male) morbidly obese patients with 36 (23 female, 13 male) normal weight controls.[9] The severely obese patients were all undergoing a laparoscopic Roux-en Y gastric bypass procedure and the normal weight controls were selected at random, although it does not say how these subjects were recruited. Nineteen GI symptoms were grouped into symptom clusters (abdominal pain, GERD, IBS, reflux, and dysphagia) and assessed using a validated questionnaire. The severely obese patients had an average BMI of 47.8 ± 4.9 kg/m^2; no average BMI is given for the normal weight control group. The mean age of the severely obese patients was 37.3 ± 8.6 years, and the normal weight subjects were 39.8 ± 11.2 years. The severely obese patients reported a significantly higher prevalence of abdominal pain ($P<.001$), GERD ($P<.001$), IBS ($P = .02$), and reflux ($P<.001$) compared with normal weight subjects. However, there was no difference in the rates of dysphagia between the 2 groups.

Delgado-Aros and Colleagues 2004

This was the first population-based study to assess GI symptoms among obese individuals.[10] This study from the United States consisted of 1963 subjects from

2660 (74% response rate) who were randomly selected to receive 2 validated questionnaires (GastroEsophageal Reflux Questionnaire [GERQ] and the Bowel Disease Questionnaire [BDQ]). The classifications of BMI included underweight, normal weight, overweight, obese class I, obese class II, and obese class III. The sample consisted of 51% women and 57% more than 50 years old. The study reported an overall increase in GI symptoms in obese individuals compared with those with normal BMI. The study found a positive relationship between BMI and frequent vomiting ($P = .02$), upper abdominal pain ($P = .03$), bloating ($P = .002$), and diarrhea ($P = .01$). Moreover, there was an increased prevalence of frequent lower abdominal pain, nausea, and constipation among obese individuals compared with normal weight subjects, but this was not statistically significant.

Talley and Colleagues 2004a

This study was conducted on a birth cohort from New Zealand aged 26 years and aimed to evaluate the association between BMI and specific GI symptoms.[11] The sample consisted of 980 individuals (94% of the original cohort), with 52.1% male. The sample completed a validated BDQ. The classifications of BMI included normal weight, overweight, and obese (BMI >30 kg/m²). There was a significant correlation between prevalence of diarrhea and increasing BMI. There was no significant correlation evident for increased BMI and the prevalence of reported abdominal pain, bloating, heartburn, acid regurgitation, constipation, or IBS.

Talley and Colleagues 2004b

This population-based study conducted in Sydney, Australia, consisted of 777 adult subjects randomly selected from the community.[12] The study evaluated the association between BMI and specific GI symptoms. The sample selected was 60% female. The mean age was not reported. Subjects completed a validated BSQ. The classifications of BMI included underweight, normal weight, overweight, and obese (BMI >30 kg/m²). Prevalence increased significantly with BMI for the following GI symptoms: increased stools ($P<.001$), loose watery stools ($P = .02$), heartburn ($P<.001$), acid regurgitation ($P = .001$). In addition, there were significant inverse relationships associated with early satiety ($P = .03$).

Aro and Colleagues 2005

The setting for this study was northern Sweden (Kalix and Haparanda) in a community-based endoscopic study of 1001 adults.[13] This study aimed to determine whether obese subjects experience more gastroesophageal reflux symptoms than normal weight subjects. Individuals were asked to complete the validated Abdominal Symptom Questionnaire (ASQ), which assessed 27 troublesome GI symptoms, and underwent an upper endoscopy. BMI was calculated at the endoscopy visit. Fifty-one percent of the subjects were women with a mean age of 53.5 years. The classifications of BMI included normal weight, overweight, and obese (BMI >30 kg/m²). Increasing BMI was associated with dysphagia, retching, acid regurgitation, vomiting, heartburn, central chest pain, burning feeling rising in chest, diarrhea, alternating constipation/diarrhea, incomplete rectal evacuation, urgency, and flatus.

Levy and Colleagues 2005

This study assessed GI symptoms among a group of obese individuals in a weight-loss program.[18] The study was conducted in the United States and included 983 participants (70% women) who had a mean age of 52.7 years. There was no other BMI category (control group) in this study. The BMI was assessed as a continuous variable. No comparisons could be made using the data from this study because the participants were involved in a weight-loss program as part of the study design.

Van Oijen and Colleagues 2006

This patient-based study from the Netherlands recruited 1023 consecutive adult patients who presented for endoscopic assessment of symptoms.[14] This study aimed to assess the relationship between BMI and GI disorders among patients referred for endoscopy. Patients were sent the validated Gastrointestinal Symptom Rating Scale (GSRS), which asks questions about 8 symptoms. The classifications of BMI included underweight, normal weight, overweight, and obese (BMI >30 kg/m^2). None of the GI symptoms showed a statistically significant association for increasing prevalence and increasing BMI. Most symptoms were consistently equal across the BMI groups, specifically for GERD, regurgitation, dyspepsia, lower abdominal pain, and heartburn. The lack of correlation between BMI groups conceivably may be caused by selection bias of a patient-population sample that was more likely to have GI symptoms, no matter what the BMI category.

Cremonini and Colleagues 2006

This prospective cohort from Olmstead County in Minnesota in the United States consisted of 637 individuals after a 10-year follow-up period.[15] This study assessed the relationship between changes in body weight and changes in upper GI symptoms. All subjects completed the BDQ, which assessed 46 GI symptoms. The classifications of BMI included underweight, normal weight, overweight, and obese (BMI >30 kg/m^2); weight change as either gain or loss during the follow-up period was determined. The study group was 53% female, mean age 62 years. Notably, an increase of 4.53 kg (10 lb) between the baseline survey and the 10-year follow-up survey was associated with new onset dyspepsia dysmotility ($P<.01$).

Cremonini and Colleagues 2009

This large population-based study included 4096 adults from the Rochester Epidemiology Project (REP) in Minnesota in the United States.[16] This study aimed to assess overeating and binge eating among various categories of BMI (underweight/normal weight and overweight/obese). All subjects completed the BDQ, which assessed 16 GI symptoms. The classifications of BMI included underweight, normal weight, overweight, and obese (BMI >30 kg/m^2). The mean age was 51 years; the gender of the population was not reported. Unfortunately, the data in this study did not allow for assessment of prevalence data and increasing BMI as these data were only reported for those classified as "no binge eating," "binge eating," or "binge eating disorder."

Pourhoseingholi and Colleagues 2009

A large cross-sectional household survey was conducted by interview in Tehran, Iran.[17] The aim of this study was to determine the relationship between BMI and functional constipation. A total of 18,180 adults were randomly sampled based on a list from the central post office. A total of 2790 individuals had at least 1 GI symptom and were included in the analysis. The classifications of BMI included normal weight, overweight, and obese (BMI >30 kg/m^2). The questionnaire consisted of 2 sections: a section asking about GI symptoms and questions based on the Rome III criteria for functional GI disorders. There were no data on age or gender for this sample; however, for a subsample of 459 individuals who were assessed for functional constipation, the mean age was 47 years and the sample consisted of 70% women. Significant trends in prevalence of GI symptoms associated with increasing BMI

Table 2
Prevalence (%) of GI symptoms among normal weight subjects

GI Symptom	Delgado-Aros et al[10]	Talley et al[11]	Talley et al[12]	Aro et al[13]	Cremonini et al[16]	Van Oijen et al[14]	Pourhoseingholi et al[17]
Abdominal distention				36.2			
Abdominal pain		13.2					41.8
Abdominal pain, upper	3.5		20.6				
Abdominal pain, lower	4.4		30.9			61.0	
Acid regurgitation		23.8	3.6	21.6		38.0	
Anal bleeding							5.6
Anal blockage							
Anal pain							13.3
Bloating	11.4	9.3	29.1				54.2
Borborygmi				28.7			
Burning feeling in chest				14.4			
Chest pain				19.2	5.9		
Constipation	16.6	20.3		25.9			40.4
Decreased stools			4.2				
Diarrhea	17.1	17.3		19.9			8.5
Dysmotility							
Dyspepsia					12.1	68.0	
Dysphagia				6.2			5.4
Early satiety			10.9	12.1			
Epigastric pain							
Fecal incontinence							1.3
Fecal urgency							
Flatus				22.2			
Food in stomach							
Frequent stools							
Fullness				16.4			
GERD					10.6	44.0	
Hard stools			9.4				
Heartburn		5.6	6.7	26.9		33.0	54.4
Incomplete evacuation				27.3			
Increased stools			23.3				
IBS		17.7					
Loose watery stools			9.7				
Lumpy hard stools							
Nausea	7.9		9.7	13.2			9.2

(continued on next page)

GI Symptom	Delgado-Aros et al[10]	Talley et al[11]	Talley et al[12]	Aro et al[13]	Cremonini et al[16]	Van Oijen et al[14]	Pourhoseingholi et al[17]
Nightly urge to defecate				5.4			
Pain at defecation				11.7			
Pain relieved by defecation				20.4			
Postprandial fullness			8.5				
Retching				21.0			
Satiety	6.5						
Straining				25.9			
Urgency				19.8			
Vomiting	1.2		2.1	2.4			9.2

included bloating ($P<.001$), incontinence ($P = .02$), heartburn ($P = .04$), nausea, and vomiting ($P = .01$). There were no associations with constipation, diarrhea, anal pain, anal bleeding, or dysphagia.

Extreme Obesity

Currently, only 2 studies have assessed GI symptoms among those classified as either obese class II (BMI 35.0–39.9 kg/m^2) or extremely obese (BMI >40 kg/m^2).[9,10] Collectively, the studies suggest that those individuals in these groups are much more likely to suffer from certain symptoms. One study[10] contained class II and class III BMI categories and prevalent symptoms included upper abdominal pain, bloating, diarrhea, and satiety, however, this study only assessed 8 symptoms abdominal pain (upper), abdominal pain (lower), bloating, constipation, diarrhea, nausea, satiety, vomiting and therefore the symptom evaluation is limited compared with other studies.

SUMMARY ANALYSIS OF REPORTED STUDIES

The studies conducted so far suggest that certain GI symptoms are more prevalent with increasing BMI (**Tables 2–4**). Collective evidence from these studies suggests that in overweight/obese patients, a large number of GI symptoms are significantly associated with increasing BMI. These include diarrhea, bloating, vomiting, abdominal pain, heartburn, flatus, constipation, straining, GERD, IBS, reflux, nausea, increased stools, loose watery stools, dysphagia, retching, central chest pain, incomplete evacuation, urgency, and dyspepsia dysmotility. Moreover, studies contradict each other for the same GI symptom (eg, dysphagia). Future analyses that break down this large collection of symptoms into a smaller and more realistic number of categoric symptoms would be useful.

Study Design and Sample

Most studies have been cross-sectional in design (7/9, 78%); 2 studies included prospective cohorts (see **Table 1**). The study samples used have been mostly population-based (community), with 2 studies using patient-based groups. Of these 2

Table 3
Prevalence (%) of GI symptoms among overweight subjects

GI symptom	Delgado-Aros et al[10]	Talley et al[11]	Talley et al[12]	Aro et al[13]	Cremonini et al[16]	Van Oijen et al[14]	Pourhoseingholi et al[17]
Abdominal distention				33.5			
Abdominal pain		9.7					39.0
Abdominal pain, upper	10.3		25.5				
Abdominal pain, lower	7.8		26.6			57.0	
Acid regurgitation		24.9	9.9	25.5		41.0	
Anal bleeding							6.8
Anal blockage							
Anal pain							15.6
Bloating	14.2	6.9	30.8				58.5
Borborygmi				30.9			
Burning feeling in chest				19.9			
Chest pain				22.0	8.0		
Constipation	17.2	17.3		21.2			38.9
Decreased stools			4.2				
Diarrhea	17.6	19.5		26.1			9.0
Dysmotility							
Dyspepsia					10.4	65.0	
Dysphagia				6.2			4.5
Early satiety			8.7	13.9			
Epigastric pain							
Fecal incontinence							1.5
Fecal urgency							
Flatus				28.6			
Food in stomach							
Frequent stools							
Fullness				18.2			
GERD					22.3	44.0	
Hard stools			10.6				
Heartburn		5.4	17.5	35.1		35.0	60.5
Incomplete evacuation				27.8			
Increased stools			27.0				
IBS		18.4					
Loose watery stools			7.6				
Lumpy hard stools							
Nausea	6.8		8.7	13.0			6.2
Nightly urge to defecate				5.5			
Pain at defecation				9.5			

(continued on next page)

Table 3
(continued)

GI symptom	Delgado-Aros et al[10]	Talley et al[11]	Talley et al[12]	Aro et al[13]	Cremonini et al[16]	Van Oijen et al[14]	Pourhoseingholi et al[17]
Pain relieved by defecation				21.2			
Postprandial fullness			12.5				
Retching				22.7			
Satiety	6.1						
Straining				22.8			
Urgency				20.8			
Vomiting	1.5		2.7	3.1			6.2

studies, 1 consisted of patients undergoing gastric bypass surgery and the other was study involved patients undergoing endoscopy. In 1 population-based study, all subjects recruited underwent endoscopy as part of the protocol.[13] There have been no patient-based studies conducted in a hospital environment.

Geographic Location

These studies were conducted in various locations around the world. The majority have been in North America (n = 4); other locations include the Pacific region (n = 2), Europe (n = 2), and the Middle East (n = 1). There have been no reported studies from Asia, Africa, United Kingdom, the Mediterranean, South America, or Russia.

Sample Size

The sample size of the studies conducted range from 43 to 4960 subjects, with a mean sample size of 1477 subjects. The studies have progressively increased in size with time. Most studies were cross-sectional in design given the logistical difficulties associated with conducting large cohort studies.

BMI Assessment

All studies used BMI as a measure of obesity. Almost all studies assessed BMI as a categorical variable with 1 study using BMI as a continuous variable.[18] The study of Foster and colleagues[9] contained only 2 BMI groups, those severely obese (BMI >40 kg/m^2) and those with a normal BMI. It is not clear in the initial study by Crowell and colleagues[8] whether BMI was determined from a questionnaire or actual measurement of weight and height in the clinic. Most population-based studies determined BMI using self-reported questionnaires.[10,12,15-17] The birth cohort study had accurate weight and height information for each individual, which was taken twice then averaged to calculate a BMI (this study also determined waist-to-hip ratio).[11] In 1 of the patient-based endoscopic studies the BMI was determined by staff who measured height and weight during the endoscopic visit[13]; the other endoscopy study collected BMI data in the form of weight and height from a questionnaire.[14] Only 2 studies assessed individuals with BMIs in obese class II[10] and obese class III.[9]

GI Symptom Assessment

All studies determined GI symptoms by self-reporting questionnaires.[8-18] Three studies used the BDQ,[10,15,16] 3 used the BSQ,[8,11,12] 1 used the GERQ,[10] 1 used the

Table 4
Prevalence (%) of GI symptoms among obese class I subjects

GI Symptom	Delgado-Aros et al[10]	Talley et al[11]	Talley et al[12]	Aro et al[13]	Cremonini et al[16]	Van Oijen et al[14]	Pourhoseingholi et al[17]
Abdominal distention				34.2			
Abdominal pain		14.7					39.3
Abdominal pain, upper	16.7		26.2				
Abdominal pain, lower	5.2		29.1			57.0	
Acid regurgitation		25.7	10.5	38.3		44.0	
Anal bleeding							6.3
Anal blockage							
Anal pain							16.7
Bloating	25.3	7.3		34.3			62.3
Borborygmi				27.0			
Burning feeling in chest				24.7			
Chest pain				26.1	12.8		
Constipation	17.0	24.8		23.8			40.7
Decreased stools			5.2				
Diarrhea	26.6	27.5		33.1			8.1
Dysmotility							
Dyspepsia					14.1	70.0	
Dysphagia				9.9			7.7
Early satiety			4.7	11.7			
Epigastric pain							
Fecal incontinence							3.3
Fecal urgency							
Flatus				28.8			
Food in stomach							
Frequent stools							
Fullness				18.4			
GERD					15.4	52.0	
Hard stools			9.9				
Heartburn		8.3	16.9	42.5		44.0	52.3
Incomplete evacuation				37.7			
Increased stools			39.0				
Irritable bowel syndrome		20.4					
Loose watery stools			18.0				
Lumpy hard stools							
Nausea	10.6		9.9	15.4			9.8
Nightly urge to defecate				12.4			

(continued on next page)

Table 4
(continued)

GI Symptom	Delgado-Aros et al[10]	Talley et al[11]	Talley et al[12]	Aro et al[13]	Cremonini et al[16]	Van Oijen et al[14]	Pourhoseingholi et al[17]
Pain at defecation				10.0			
Pain relieved by defecation				20.5			
Postprandial fullness			8.1				
Retching				32.7			
Satiety	9.8						
Straining				24.7			
Urgency				28.6			
Vomiting	3.0		2.9	6.2		9.8	

ASQ,[13] 1 used the GSRS,[14] and 2 used unknown instruments that were not described.[9,18] One of these studies did describe the use of a Rome III questionnaire but it is unclear if the data obtained on GI symptoms were from this instrument.[18]

FUTURE STUDIES: NEW QUESTIONS AND DIRECTIONS

The studies aiming to determine the epidemiology and relationship between GI symptoms and the body weight categories of overweight, obese, and extremely obese have provided a rich pool of data. Based on the findings and methodologies used, researchers have the opportunity to learn from these studies. However, several questions arise from analysis of the studies reported to date. 1. Should standardized questionnaires be used to obtain a broad range of GI symptoms rather than just a few suspected key GI symptoms? 2. Are self-reported weight and height data accurate and reliable in population-based studies? 3. What potential confounders should be adjusted for in theses analyses? 4. Are there statistical interactions that could be assessed, such as gene/environment, carbohydrate/fat, insulin resistance, food/disease interactions? 5. Do community-based studies provide a more precise picture of the epidemiology of GI symptoms and BMI than patient-based groups (patients recruited for studies from a clinical practice setting such as a hospital who may be more likely to have increased symptoms anyway)? 6. Do obese children have the same GI symptoms as obese adults? These are just some of the questions that require further clarification as this important area of GI research develops.

Additional studies from various geographic locations around the world will greatly enhance the pool of studies and should provide insight into cultural, behavioral, and even physiologic disparities among those with increased BMI who have more GI symptoms than those of normal weight. Moreover, the relationship between increasing BMI and conditions such as IBS should be further investigated in separate studies with adequate adjustment for potential confounders. Because of the dearth of studies assessing those with class II obesity (BMI 35.0–39.9 kg/m^2) and extreme obesity (BMI >40 kg/m^2), further research into the role of GI symptoms is urgently required among these groups, and should include the assessment of a greater number of GI symptoms in well-designed and adequately statistically powered studies. The response to weight reduction and the response of these symptoms to thresholds for weight loss will be a fertile area of research of particular interest in assessing medical and surgical therapies for weight reduction. There is much yet to be learned as we develop and best define the appropriate management strategies to optimize the short- and long-term clinical outcomes for obese and overweight patients.

REFERENCES

1. Brawer R, Brisbon N, Plumb J. Obesity and cancer. Prim Care Clin Office Pract 2009;36:509–31.
2. Allison KC, Stunkard AJ. Obesity and eating disorders. Psychiatr Clin North Am 2005;28:55–67.
3. Li Z, Bowerman S, Heber D. Health ramifications of the obesity epidemic. Surg Clin North Am 2005;85:681–701.
4. Shah MB. Obesity and sexuality in women. Obstet Gynecol Clin North Am 2009; 36:347–60.
5. Yogev Y, Catalano PM. Pregnancy and obesity. Obstet Gynecol Clin North Am 2009;36:285–300.
6. Flegal KM, Carroll MD, Ogden CL, et al. Prevalence and trends in obesity among US adults, 1999–2000. JAMA 2002;288:1723–7.
7. Ogden CL, Carroll MD, Curtin LR, et al. Prevalence of overweight and obesity in the United States, 1999–2004. JAMA 2006;295:1549–55.
8. Crowell MD, Cheskin LJ, Musial F. Prevalence of gastrointestinal symptoms in obese and normal weight binge eaters. Am J Gastroenterol 1994;89:387–91.
9. Foster A, Richards WO, McDowell J, et al. Gastrointestinal symptoms are more intense in morbidly obese patients. Surg Endosc 2003;17:1766–8.
10. Delgado-Aros S, Locke GR III, Camilleri MC, et al. Obesity is associated with increased risk of gastrointestinal symptoms: a population-based study. Am J Gastroenterol 2004;99:1801–6.
11. Talley NJ, Howell S, Poulton R. Obesity and chronic gastrointestinal tract symptoms in young adults: a birth cohort study. Am J Gastroenterol 2004a;99: 1807–14.
12. Talley NJ, Quan C, Jones MP, et al. Association of upper and lower gastrointestinal tract symptoms with body mass index in an Australian cohort. Neurogastroenterol Motil 2004b;16:413–9.
13. Aro P, Ronkainen J, Talley NJ, et al. Body mass index and chronic unexplained gastrointestinal symptoms: an adult endoscopic population based study. Gut 2005;54:1377–83.
14. van Oijen MG, Josemanders DF, Laheij RJ, et al. Gastrointestinal disorders and symptoms: does body mass index matter? Neth J Med 2006;64:45–9.
15. Cremonini F, Locke GR, Schleck CD, et al. Relationship between upper gastrointestinal symptoms and changes in body weight in a population-based cohort. Neurogastroenterol Motil 2006;18:987–94.
16. Cremonini F, Camilleri M, Clark MM, et al. Associations among binge eating behavior patterns and gastrointestinal symptoms: a population-based study. Int J Obes 2009;33:342–53.
17. Pourhoseingholi MA, Kaboli SA, Pourhoseingholi A, et al. Obesity and functional constipation: a community-based study in Iran. J Gastrointestin Liver Dis 2009; 18:151–5.
18. Levy R, Linde JA, Feld KA, et al. The association of gastrointestinal symptoms with weight, diet, and exercise in weight-loss program participants. Clin Gastroenterol Hepatol 2005;3:992–6.

Gastrointestinal Symptoms and Diseases Related to Obesity: An Overview

Amy E. Foxx-Orenstein, DO

KEYWORDS

• Obesity • GI symptoms • Gut hormone • Appetite regulation

Obesity is a leading cause of illness and death worldwide.[1,2] It is one of the greatest public health challenges of this century, with more than 1.6 billion adults classified as being overweight and 400 million as obese.[3] From 1980 to 2002, rates of obesity more than doubled in the United States, reaching 32% in the adult population, thus achieving the highest rates of obesity in the developed world.[4] Although overall obesity rates began to plateau in the 2000s, severe obesity in adults and children has continued to increase.[5] The most dramatic increases have occurred in class III obesity (body mass index [BMI] ≥40), with an increase from 0.78% in 1990 to 2.2% in 2000.[5]

As the rates of obesity have escalated, it is more than just waistbands that have expanded. Obesity is a risk factor for some of the most prevalent diseases in North America, including coronary artery disease, stroke, diabetes mellitus, hypertension, and osteoarthritis.[6] Moreover, common digestive disorders, such as gastroesophageal reflux, esophagitis, nonalcoholic fatty liver, gallstones, and certain cancers, arise with greater frequency in obese individuals compared with normal-weight individuals (**Table 1**).[7]

Obesity-related health care costs have also ballooned. Americans who are obese now make up a quarter of the population and are responsible for a 40 billion-dollar rise in annual medical spending.[8] On average, an obese person spends more than 1400 dollars for his or her medical care annually, almost 42% more than is spent by a nonobese person.[8] Although there are no current recommendations for testing in the absence of symptoms or preexisting laboratory abnormalities, weight loss is a recommended strategy to prevent the symptoms that are related to obesity-related gastrointestinal disorders and to decrease the risk of progression of diseases.[7]

Division of Gastroenterology and Hepatology, Mayo Clinic College of Medicine, 200 First Street SW, Rochester, MN 55905, USA
E-mail address: Foxx-Orenstein.Amy@mayo.edu

Gastroenterol Clin N Am 39 (2010) 23–37
doi:10.1016/j.gtc.2009.12.006
0889-8553/10/$ – see front matter © 2010 Published by Elsevier Inc.

Table 1
Obesity and the risk of digestive disorders

	Magnitude of Increased Risk with Obesity (Compared with Normal or Low BMI)	Comments
Esophagus		
GERD symptoms	50%	
Erosive esophagitis	50%–100%	
Barrett esophagus	2-fold	Abdominal obesity
Adenocarcinoma	2-fold	
Gallbladder		
Stones	2- to 3-fold	More in women
Cancer	35%–85%	More in women
Pancreas		
Worse acute pancreatitis	20%–50%	
Cancer	35%–85%	Abdominal obesity
Colon		
Adenoma	50%–100%	
Cancer	2-fold	Colon (not rectum), more in men, more with abdominal obesity, postmenopausal women
Liver		
Nonalcoholic fatty liver disease	2- to 4-fold	Abdominal obesity
Advanced HCV-related disease	50%	
Cirrhosis	30%–50%	
Hepatocellular carcinoma	17%–89%	

Abbreviations: BMI, body mass index; HCV, hepatitis C virus.
  Data from American College of Gastroenterology. Obesity and digestive disorders. A physician reference, 2008. Available at: http://www.acg.gi.org/obesity/pdfs/ACG_Obesity_Physician_Reference.pdf.

GASTROINTESTINAL SYMPTOMS RELATED TO OBESITY AND OBESITY TREATMENTS

Generally defined as a BMI of 30 kg/m^2 or more (less accurate in body builders and pregnant women), obesity has been linked to a wide range of gastrointestinal symptoms.[9–12] Disruption of mechanisms that regulate appetite and satiety is fundamental to the development of obesity.[9] Acid regurgitation, heartburn, and diarrhea are some symptoms that are reported with increased frequency in obese subjects compared with normal-weight subjects (**Table 2**).[13] Pharmacologic and surgical treatments of obesity, by altering gastrointestinal function through mechanisms that regulate hunger, food intake, or absorption of nutrients, influence the energy consumed and meal termination.[14–17]

GUT HORMONES AND REGULATION OF APPETITE AND SATIETY

There are 3 primary mechanisms that control appetite: 1) the hypothalamus serves as the center for the integration of feeding and associated neuroendocrine and

Table 2
Odds for symptom reporting in overweight and obese subjects

Symptoms	Overweight OR[a]	95% CI	Obese OR[a]	95% CI
Upper gastrointestinal symptoms				
Abdominal pain	0.90	(0.66, 1.23)	1.29	(0.93, 1.78)
Fullness	0.90	(0.55, 1.46)	0.89	(0.52, 1.53)
Food staying in the stomach	1.37	(0.91, 2.07)	1.76	(1.15, 2.7)
Bloating	0.98	(0.73, 1.33)	1.07	(0.77, 1.48)
Acid regurgitation	2.00	(1.39, 2.86)	3.39	(2.36, 4.87)
Heartburn	1.64	(1.16, 2.31)	3.11	(2.20, 4.39)
Nausea	0.70	(0.35, 1.40)	1.46	(0.77, 2.75)
Vomiting	1.05	(0.59, 1.87)	1.70	(0.96, 3.02)
Dysphagia	0.53	(0.30, 0.95)	0.66	(0.36, 1.18)
Lower gastrointestinal symptoms				
Anal blockage	0.63	(0.41, 0.99)	0.74	(0.46, 1.17)
Diarrhea	1.35	(0.97, 1.88)	1.64	(1.16, 2.32)
Constipation	0.72	(0.47, 1.11)	0.50	(0.30, 0.85)
Lumpy/hard stools	0.99	(0.72, 1.37)	0.49	(0.33, 0.75)
Loose/watery stools	1.09	(0.78, 1.53)	1.63	(1.15, 2.29)
Fecal urgency	1.09	(0.77, 1.54)	1.46	(1.03, 2.09)
Fecal incontinence	0.98	(0.66, 1.46)	1.36	(0.91, 2.04)

Abbreviations: CI, confidence interval; OR, odds ratio.

[a] Odds ratio (95% CI) from logistic regression model adjusting for age, gender, binge-eating category, physical activity score, and version of the survey; relative to normal weight.

Data from Cremonini M, Camilleri M, Clark MM, et al. Associations among binge eating behavior patterns and gastrointestinal symptoms: a population-based study. Int J Obes 2009;33(3):342–53.

gastrointestinal activities; 2) the gastrointestinal tract provides a rich source of hunger and satiety factors that modulate meal intake and termination[9,18]; and 3) adipose-derived leptin is involved in the long-term regulation of energy intake and expenditure.[19–21]

The gastrointestinal tract is the largest endocrine organ in the body. Gut hormones exert exocrine actions, regulate the secretion of insulin, and central nervous system circuits that control food intake, and influence gut motility.[22] They interact with the brain via the gut-brain axis through which they modulate peptide neurotransmitter release via hypothalamic and brainstem centers (**Fig. 1**). Apart from ghrelin, most gut peptides known to influence appetite, including insulin,[23] glucagon-like peptide 1 (GLP-1),[24] peptide YY (PYY),[25] oxyntomodulin (OXM),[26] cholecystokinin (CCK),[27,28] and pancreatic polypeptide (PP),[29] do so by inducing satiety and some also by affecting intestinal motility.

Ghrelin, a hormone that is synthesized primarily in the epithelial P/D1 cells of the gastric fundus,[18,30,31] is an agonist of the growth hormone receptor and a member of the motilin-related family of regulatory peptides. Ghrelin stimulates appetite and induces a positive energy balance, thus leading to body-weight gain in addition to its ability to stimulate growth hormone secretion and to accelerate gastric motility.[18] Ghrelin modulates the synthesis and secretion of several neuropeptides in the hypothalamus that stimulate feeding and regulate related hypothalamic functions.[18] Unique among gut hormones, plasma ghrelin levels gradually increase with fasting and decrease immediately after a meal, supporting a role in meal initiation.[18,32,33] Plasma ghrelin levels also increase with diet-induced weight loss,[34,35] which suggests that ghrelin may act to counter diet-induced weight loss by invigorating hunger and increasing energy intake.

Insulin is secreted by the Islets of Langerhans in the pancreas to promote storage of energy; its circulation is increased in response to food intake and in states of obesity.[36] Insulin receptors are expressed in the CNS[37] and injections of insulin into the brain of insulin-deficient animals can markedly reduce eating behavior.[38] Adipocyte-derived

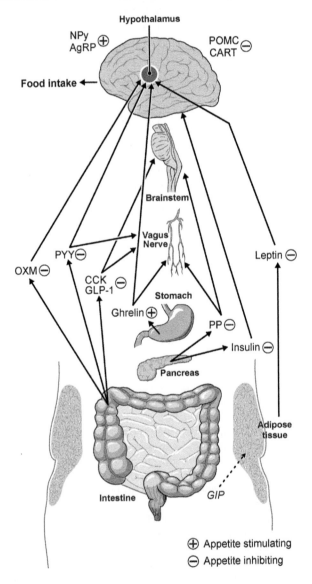

3026550-01.ai

leptin an important anorexigenic hormone that like insulin, is involved in long-term energy homeostasis. Leptin is secreted in response to a positive energy balance, and circulated to the hypothalamus and other regions of the brain inducing negative feedback responses.[39,40] The actions of ghrelin and leptin are complimentary, yet they are antagonistic in that they modulate appetite, gastric motility, and body weight by counterregulating the same hypothalamic signals, neuropeptide Y (NPY) and agouti-related peptide (AgRP). NPY and AgRP are two extremely potent orexigenic peptides of the arcuate nucleus (AR) within the hypothalamus that together act to reduce energy expenditure.[18,41–43] In addition to the inhibition of orexigenic neurons within the AR, leptin also stimulates the activity of proopiomelanocortin (POMC) and cocaine- and amphetamine-regulated transcript (CART), two anorexigenic hypothalamic neurons that contribute to increased thermogenesis and energy expenditure.[44–46] Within the AR these anatomically distinct neuronal populations provide overlapping projections to other key parts of the hypothalamus implicated in the control of feeding. As a therapeutic agent, leptin held great promise. However, exogenous administration of supraphysiologic doses of leptin failed to produce any notable diminution in appetite or weight loss.[47] To date, obesity-related resistance to the action of leptin has limited its therapeutic effectiveness.[48]

GLP-1, which is coreleased postprandially with PPY and OXM from L cells of the small intestine in proportion to the amount of energy consumed, acts as a powerful incretin, enhancing meal-related insulin secretion.[49] Clinically, long-acting GLP-1 receptor agonists (such as exendin-4) facilitate glucose control by several different mechanisms, promote a subtle yet prolonged satiety effect, and improve glycemic control when used as adjunctive therapy in patients with type 2 diabetes receiving metformin.[50] GLP-1 has been shown to delay gastric emptying and intestinal transit time.[49] Gastrointestinal inhibitory peptide (GIP), another incretin peptide, is secreted from K cells in the duodenum and proximal jejunum in the presence of glucose and fat within minutes of food ingestion.[22] Although GIP promotes energy storage through direct action on adipose tissue, it is not known to have an effect on food intake.[22]

Fig. 1. Appetite regulation via the gut-brain-leptin axis. Anorexigenic signals (−) and orexigenic signals (+). Neurons within the hypothalamus mediate many of the metabolic effects of leptin and peripheral gut hormones. NPY and AgRP are orexigenic neurons co-localized in the hypothalamus; a separate region expresses the anorexigenic neurons POMC and CART. Ghrelin is released from the stomach preprandially stimulating food intake through signals to the vagus nerve and hypothalamus. Insulin, secreted from the pancreas in response to feeding to promote energy storage reduces food intake by central mechanisms. Leptin is secreted by fat cells signaling body energy stores and downregulates feeding behavior through a variety of neural and endocrine mechanisms. PP is released from the pancreas postprandially and acts to reduce food intake through signals to the brainstem or vagus nerve. OXM, PYY, CCK, and GLP-1 are released from the intestine postprandially and can reduce food intake through signals to the hypothalamus, brainstem, and vagus nerve. GIP is released from the intestine postprandially with an anabolic effect on adipose tissue but without known effect on appetite. AgRP, agouti-related peptide; AP, area postrema; ARC, arcuate nucleus; CART, cocaine-and amphetamine-regulated transcript; CCK, cholecystokinin; GIP, gastric inhibitory polypeptide; GLP-1, glucagon-like peptide 1; NPY, neuropeptide Y; NTS, nucleus tractus solitarius; OXM, oxyntomodulin; POMC, proopiomelanocortin; PP, pancreatic polypeptide; PYY, peptide YY. (*Adapted from* Vincent RP, Ashrafian H, le Roux CW. Mechanisms of disease: the role of gastrointestinal hormones in appetite and obesity. Nat Clin Pract Gastroenterol Hepatol 2008;5(5):268–77; with permission.)

PYY3-36, the major form of PYY, reduces acute food intake in normal-weight humans[16] by modulating appetite circuits in the hypothalamus. PYY has high affinity for the Y2 family of receptors of the hypothalamus, and it inhibits orexiant NPY neurons, activates anorexiant POMC neurons and α-MSH hormone, and may contribute to its anorectic effect through actions on the vagus and brainstem.[16,25,51] The physiologic effects of PYY3-36 include delayed gastric emptying and reduced gastric secretion, and PYY has been implicated as a major constituent of the ileal brake.[3,52]

Digestion of lipids results in the release of PP, the amount secreted being proportional to the calorie content of the meal.[53] PP is considered a long-term appetite suppressant with peripheral administration in obese mice, resulting in reduced food intake and slowed weight gain.[53] The mechanism that mediates PP satiety effect remains unknown, although it is known to stimulate the Y2 receptors in the hypothalamus and may directly activate neurons in regions of the AR.[22] The actions of OXM are to diminish gastric secretion and reduce food intake when administered centrally to rodents or peripherally to rodents or humans.[26,54] OXM increases energy expenditure by more than 25% and reduces food intake, body weight, and adiposity in rodents.[55] A discrete receptor for OXM has not been identified, yet OXM does bind to the GLP-1 receptor and has been shown to cause similar patterns of central neuronal activation after peripheral administration.[56]

The anorexiant effect of CCK was recognized more than 30 years ago.[57] CCK is synthesized by L cells of the small intestine and secreted in the proximal duodenum. CCK-1 receptors are primarily expressed by vagal afferent neurons, the targets by which CCK is thought to produce the sensation of satiety.[58] The half-life of CCK is just 1 to 2 minutes, suggesting it may serve as a short-term regulator of appetite. Animal studies have shown administration of CCK to reduce food intake but increase meal frequency without affecting the body weight.[59] Biologic functions of CCK include delayed gastric emptying, stimulation of pancreatic enzyme secretion, and gallbladder contraction.[60,61]

Circulating levels of these gut hormones and those of the central nervous system can be affected by increased or decreased adiposity, pharmacotherapy, and gastrointestinal bypass surgery.

EFFECT OF OBESITY TREATMENTS ON GASTROINTESTINAL SYMPTOMS

Of the two Food and Drug Administration–approved medications for the long-term treatment of obesity, sibutramine acts as anorexiant, whereas orlistat impairs the digestion and absorption of dietary fat.[14] Anorexiants increase satiation (level of fullness or meal-related satisfaction), which regulates the amount of food consumed or the level of satiety (absence of hunger) and determines the frequency of eating.[62] Sibutramine is a centrally acting serotonin and noradrenaline reuptake inhibitor that inhibits appetite and induces thermogenesis, thus contributing to reduced energy intake with enhanced energy expenditure.[63] Predictably, fat malabsorption that occurs with the use of orlistat results in oily and frequent bowel movements, fecal urgency, and flatulence. With continued use, deficiencies in the fat-soluble vitamins A, D, E, and K may occur.[64]

All surgeries that restrict gastric luminal capacity cause satiety when solid food is ingested, leading to reduced calorie intake and loss of weight.[65] Nausea, bloating, and vomiting are common after bypass surgery owing to restricted anatomy and altered motility.[65] These symptoms may subside with increased fluid intake, reduced food volume, chewing food well, and slow eating, although testing to exclude dehydration or a complication of surgery may be warranted if symptoms persist. Small intestine bacterial overgrowth is a frequent late complication of gastric bypass, as established by elevated serum folate levels and detection of abnormal glucose-hydrogen breath testing.[66–68] Symptoms of bacterial overgrowth may include abdominal bloating, nausea, abdominal cramping and discomfort, steatorrhea, flatulence, anemia, and weight loss.

Gastric bypass can result in dumping syndrome when high-density carbohydrates are consumed.[69] Early dumping symptoms comprise both gastrointestinal (nausea, vomiting, abdominal pain, diarrhea and bloating) and vasomotor symptoms, whereas late dumping symptoms are the results of reactive hypoglycemia.[70] Rapid gastric emptying that delivers a significant proportion of nutrients quickly to the small intestine as well as large, difficult-to-digest particles contributes to the pathogenesis of this syndrome. The result is a fluid shift from the intravascular component to the intestinal lumen, which results in cardiovascular symptoms, release of several gastrointestinal and pancreatic hormones, and late postprandial hypoglycemia.[70] Nutrient diversion into the distal small intestine causes iron and B12 deficiency anemia and thiamine deficiency[71] and may also worsen lactose intolerance. After gastric bypass, patients may experience constipation caused by decreased food or water intake, or in some patients, iron supplementation, narcotics, or antidepressants.[72] They may also experience diarrhea that can be related to dietary fat. Reduced fat intake or supplementation of a small amount of pancreatic enzymes may reduce symptoms. With rapid weight loss, there is an increased risk for developing gallstones. About 1 in 10 people with gastric bypass will experience problems from gallstones and will need their gallbladders to be removed.[73] In the postbariatric setting, additional gastrointestinal symptom–related problems may include intestinal obstruction, migration of mechanical devices (vertical banded gastroplasty), fistula formation, disruption of suture lines, and chronic nutritional deficiencies (malabsorption) associated with a range of gastrointestinal complaints.[69,74]

EFFECT OF BARIATRIC SURGERY ON GUT HORMONES

Gastric bypass is a surgical technique that combines gastric restriction with bypass of the stomach to variable lengths of the small intestine that leads to significant, sustained weight loss in patients with severe obesity.[75,76] Small gastric pouch size is a key determinant in the early satiation and persistently suppressed appetite that occurs after this type of surgery.[77,78] Malabsorption does not appear to play as large a role in weight loss after a short-limb intestinal bypass compared with that played after long-limb bypass.[76] Yet, as bypass surgery seems to be more beneficial in achieving sustained weight loss than purely restrictive gastric surgery, it was hypothesized that interference in other factors affecting energy balance may add to the effectiveness of this type of surgery.[78,79] Roux-en-Y gastric bypass has been shown to cause a decline in plasma ghrelin levels in most subjects[32,34,41,80] and a distinct increase in GLP-1 and PYY plasma levels compared with gastric banding and control patients,[78] possibly contributing to the significant and lasting weight-reducing effects of the procedure.[78,80] In patients experiencing poor weight loss after gastric bypass procedures, the postprandial PYY and GLP-1 responses were attenuated compared with patients with good postoperative weight loss.[81] Inhibiting the satiety gut hormone responses with octreotide after successful RYGB resulted in the return of appetite and increase in food intake.[81,82] It seems that bariatric surgery provides a stimulus to the distal small intestine mucosal endocrine L cells, resulting in an increase in PYY, GLP-1, and many of the enteroglucagon family of gut peptides.[81,82]

Laparoscopic adjustable gastric banding surgery involves the creation of a small gastric pouch by securing a modifiable restrictive gastric band just below the gastro-esophageal junction.[83] The band can be adjusted to achieve desired weight and nutritional outcomes. In a randomized controlled trial that compared optimal with lesser gastric band restriction, optimal restriction was associated with greater fasting and postprandial satiety levels ($P<.01$), whereas plasma ghrelin, leptin, and insulin levels did not change between optimal and reduced restriction and were not significantly different from normal levels.[83]

Overall, gut hormones that are affected by bypassing the stomach and proximal small intestine and by enhanced nutrient delivery to the distal intestine may play a major role in mediating weight loss after gastric bypass.[84,85]

GASTROINTESTINAL SYMPTOMS ASSOCIATED WITH INCREASED BMI

Several studies have demonstrated an association between obesity and gastrointestinal symptoms.[9,10,86,87] In a population-based study, acid regurgitation, heartburn, food staying in the stomach, vomiting, nausea, upper abdominal pain, bloating, and diarrhea occurred more often in obese patients with binge-eating disorders (see **Table 2**).[13] In this study, an increase in body weight of more than 4.5 kg during a 10-year period was associated with the onset of new gastrointestinal symptoms.[13] BMI is an independent risk factor for the presence of self-reported heartburn, regurgitation, and bloating in a United States community-based population.[9]

In a meta-analysis, Nguyen and El-Serag[88] showed that a high BMI was associated with an increased risk of heartburn, regurgitation, and water brash compared with a normal BMI. Overweight and obesity have been shown to be the strong independent risk factors of gastroesophageal reflux disease (GERD) symptoms and erosive esophagitis,[89] with the suggestion of a dose-response relationship.

GASTROINTESTINAL DISEASES RELATED TO OBESITY

Obesity has been shown to be a risk factor for many gastrointestinal disorders (see **Table 1**).[7]

Obesity and the Esophagus

An increase in the prevalence of obesity and GERD in Western populations during the past 50 years suggests that an association exists between these 2 conditions, with most epidemiologic studies supporting this conclusion.[90] Clinical trials that examined the relationship of increased BMI and GERD-related disorders found that a high BMI was associated with a 1.5- to 2.5-fold increase in the risk of GERD and its complications, including symptoms of heartburn and regurgitation, erosive esophagitis, and esophageal adenocarcinoma.[91,92] In a recent meta-analysis, increased BMI was strongly associated with esophageal adenocarcinoma in men (relative risk of 1.52, $P<.0001$) and in women (1.51, $P<.0001$).[93] Abdominal diameter but not BMI is associated with a 2-fold increased risk of developing Barrett esophagus (BE).[94–96] Obesity is only an indirect risk factor for developing BE, with BMI status having no predictive value with respect to the progression of symptoms to BE.[97] Truncal obesity poses a higher risk for developing BE in male Caucasians than peripheral obesity.[88,94] Anatomic and physiologic obesity-related changes, including reduced lower esophageal sphincter pressure, presence of a hiatal hernia, increased intragastric pressure, and esophageal motility disorders, may account for some of the findings.[90]

Obesity and the Gallbladder

In the general population, immutable risk factors for developing gallstones are female gender, increased age, and genetic traits. Obesity, the metabolic syndrome, and rapid weight loss are the modifiable risk factors of gallstone formation.[98] After bariatric surgery, traditional risk factors are not predictive of symptomatic gallstone formation. Weight loss of more than 25% of original weight postoperatively was the only predictive factor for the development of gallstones and selection of patients for subsequent cholecystectomy.[99] A meta-analysis of prospective observational studies showed that a 5-kg/m^2 increase in BMI was strongly associated with gallbladder cancer in women (1.59, P = .04) but not in men (1.09, P = .12).[93]

Obesity and the Liver

The prevalence of nonalcoholic fatty liver disease (NAFLD), cirrhosis, and hepatocellular carcinoma has been independently associated with obesity,[88] with the correlation between fatty liver and obesity being particularly strong.[100] In the general population, the prevalence of NAFLD ranges from 3% to 24% but increases to 58% to 74% in obese subjects.[88] Obesity is frequently accompanied by the metabolic syndrome, a persistent inflammatory state that promotes fatty acid accumulation as it promotes insulin resistance.[101] As the severity of the metabolic syndrome worsens, the risk of developing liver damage, such as nonalcoholic steatohepatitis (NASH), increases. Severe NASH is an uncommon complication of NAFLD, but it was reported in some obese patients after jejunoileal bypass surgery, characterized by sudden onset of fever, jaundice, and tender hepatomegaly and associated with a flu-like prodrome.[102,103] The progressive liver disease that developed in conjunction with this surgical technique led to the abandonment of the procedure as a means of weight loss.[102] NASH is an uncommon complication of modern bypass surgery.[104] Autopsy series have shown a 6-fold increase in the relative risk of developing cirrhosis in obesity.[105] The risk of developing hepatocellular carcinoma is also increased.[88,106] A meta-analysis of overweight and obesity relative to liver cancer showed in summary results that the risk was 17 and 89% higher, respectively, compared with those of normal weight.[106] The relative risk of hepatic cancer was considerably higher in men (2.42) compared with that in women (1.67).

Obesity and the Colon

Increased adiposity seems to be a risk factor for developing adenocarcinoma of the colon and adenomatous polyps. A large meta-analysis by Ansary Moghaddam and colleagues[107] showed a relative risk of colorectal cancer of 1.19 (95% confidence interval [CI], 1.11–1.29) when comparing obese individuals with normal-weight individuals and a relative risk of 1.45 (95% CI, 1.31–1.61) when comparing those with a high central adiposity measure with those with a low measure. The risk of developing colon cancer in women was lower (1.08; 95% CI, 0.98–1.18) than that in men (1.41; 95% CI, 1.30–1.54). The BMI-related risk of colon cancer was higher and less evident in young women than in older women. There was a dose-response relationship between colorectal cancer and BMI, in which for every 2-kg/m^2 increase in BMI, the risk of colorectal cancer increased by 7% and for a 2-cm increase in waist circumference, the risk increased by 4%.[88] In a separate study, obesity was found to be a risk factor for advanced adenomatous polyps. For every 1-unit increase in BMI more than 30, there was a corresponding 1% increase in the frequency of advanced adenomas.[108]

SUMMARY

There is a clear relationship between obesity and many gastrointestinal symptoms. Appetite and satiety are symptoms that are highly regulated through a neuroendocrine, gut-brain-adipose axis. Diet, pharmacologic, and surgical approaches to lose weight are influenced by this complex, redundant neuroendocrine regulatory system. Obesity increases the risk of many digestive disorders, including many cancers. Some unresolved issues relate to what appropriate measure of adiposity is used in terms of disease risk, the mechanisms that underlie gender differences, and the effect of weight loss on specific disease-related risks. Knowledge of these issues will provide the basis to develop health strategies to prevent obesity-related diseases.

REFERENCES

1. Kopelman PG. Obesity as a medical problem. Nature 2000;404(6778):635–43.
2. Lew EA. Mortality and weight: insured lives and the American Cancer Society studies. Ann Intern Med 1985;103(6 Pt 2):1024–9.
3. Karra E, Chandarana K, Batterham RL. The role of peptide YY in appetite regulation and obesity. J Physiol 2009;587(Pt 1):19–25.
4. Ogden CL, Carroll MD, Curtin LR, et al. Prevalence of overweight and obesity in the United States, 1999–2004. JAMA 2006;295(13):1549–55.
5. Freedman DS, Khan LK, Serdula MK, et al. Trends and correlates of class 3 obesity in the United States from 1990 through 2000. JAMA 2002;288(14):1758–61.
6. Field AE, Coakley EH, Must A, et al. Impact of overweight on the risk of developing common chronic diseases during a 10-year period. Arch Intern Med 2001;161(13):1581–6.
7. American College of Gastroenterology. Obesity and digestive disorders. A physician reference. 2008. Available at: www.acg.gi.org/obesity/pdfs/ACG_Obesity_Physician_Reference.pdf. Accessed December 2, 2009.
8. Finkelstein EA, Trogdon JG, Cohen JW, et al. Annual medical spending attributable to obesity: payer- and service-specific estimates. Health Aff 2009;28(5):w822–31.
9. Delgado-Aros S, Locke GR 3rd, Camilleri M, et al. Obesity is associated with increased risk of gastrointestinal symptoms: a population-based study. Am J Gastroenterol 2004;99(9):1801–6.
10. Crowell MD, Cheskin LJ, Musial F. Prevalence of gastrointestinal symptoms in obese and normal weight binge eaters. Am J Gastroenterol 1994;89(3):387–91.
11. Pourhoseingholi MA, Kaboli SA, Pourhoseingholi A, et al. Obesity and functional constipation; a community-based study in Iran. J Gastrointestin Liver Dis 2009;18(2):151–5.
12. Ayazi S, Hagen J, Chan L, et al. Obesity and gastroesophageal reflux: quantifying the association between body mass index, esophageal acid exposure, and lower esophageal sphincter status in a large series of patients with reflux symptoms. J Gastrointest Surg 2009;13(8):1440–7.
13. Cremonini F, Camilleri M, Clark MM, et al. Associations among binge eating behavior patterns and gastrointestinal symptoms: a population-based study. Int J Obes 2009;33(3):342–53.
14. Czernichow S, Lee CMY, Barzi F, et al. Efficacy of weight loss drugs on obesity and cardiovascular risk factors in obese adolescents: a meta-analysis of randomized controlled trials. Obes Rev 2009, July 1. [Epub ahead of print].

15. Roux C, Aylwin S, Batterham R, et al. Gut hormone profiles following bariatric surgery favor an anorectic state, facilitate weight loss, and improve metabolic parameters. Ann Surg 2006;243(1):108–14.
16. Batterham RL, Cohen MA, Ellis SM, et al. Inhibition of food intake in obese subjects by peptide YY3-36. N Engl J Med 2003;349(10):941–8.
17. Gutzwiller J-P, Hruz P, Huber AR, et al. Glucagon-like peptide-1 is involved in sodium and water homeostasis in humans. Digestion 2006;73(2–3):142–50.
18. Inui A, Asakawa A, Bowers CY, et al. Ghrelin, appetite, and gastric motility: the emerging role of the stomach as an endocrine organ. FASEB J 2004;18(3):439–56.
19. Williams KW, Scott MM, Elmquist JK. From observation to experimentation: leptin action in the mediobasal hypothalamus. Am J Clin Nutr 2009;89(3): 985S–90S.
20. Schwartz MW, Morton GJ. Obesity: keeping hunger at bay. Nature 2002; 418(6898):595–7.
21. Schwartz M, Woods S, Porte D Jr, et al. Central nervous system control of food intake. Nature 2000;404:661–71.
22. Vincent RP, Ashrafian H, le Roux CW. Mechanisms of disease: the role of gastrointestinal hormones in appetite and obesity. Nat Clin Pract Gastroenterol Hepatol 2008;5(5):268–77.
23. Pliquett RU, Fuhrer D, Falk S, et al. The effects of insulin on the central nervous system–focus on appetite regulation. Horm Metab Res 2006;38(7):442–6.
24. Lovshin JA, Drucker DJ. Glucagon-like peptides, the central nervous system, and the regulation of energy homeostasis. Curr Med Chem Cent Nerv Syst Agents 2003;3(2):73–80.
25. Batterham RL, Cowley MA, Small CJ, et al. Gut hormone PYY (3-36) physiologically inhibits food intake. Nature 2002;418(6898):650–4.
26. Cohen MA, Ellis SM, Le Roux CW, et al. Oxyntomodulin suppresses appetite and reduces food intake in humans. J Clin Endocrinol Metab 2003;88(10): 4696–701.
27. Barrachina MD, Martinez V, Wang L, et al. Synergistic interaction between leptin and cholecystokinin to reduce short-term food intake in lean mice. Proc Natl Acad Sci U S A 1997;94(19):10455–60.
28. Moran TH, Ameglio PJ, Schwartz GJ, et al. Blockade of type A, not type B, CCK receptors attenuates satiety actions of exogenous and endogenous CCK. Am J Physiol 1992;262(1 Pt 2):R46–50.
29. Asakawa A, Inui A, Yuzuriha H, et al. Characterization of the effects of pancreatic polypeptide in the regulation of energy balance. Gastroenterology 2003; 124(5):1325–36.
30. Nakazato M, Murakami N, Date Y, et al. A role for ghrelin in the central regulation of feeding. Nature 2001;409(6817):194–8.
31. Wren AM, Seal LJ, Cohen MA, et al. Ghrelin enhances appetite and increases food intake in humans. J Clin Endocrinol Metab 2001;86(12):5992.
32. Cummings DE, Purnell JQ, Frayo RS, et al. A preprandial rise in plasma ghrelin levels suggests a role in meal initiation in humans. Diabetes 2001; 50(8):1714–9.
33. Date Y, Kojima M, Hosoda H, et al. Ghrelin, a novel growth hormone-releasing acylated peptide, is synthesized in a distinct endocrine cell type in the gastrointestinal tracts of rats and humans. Endocrinology 2000;141(11):4255–61.
34. Cummings DE, Weigle DS, Frayo RS, et al. Plasma ghrelin levels after diet-induced weight loss or gastric bypass surgery. N Engl J Med 2002;346(21): 1623–30.

35. Hansen TK, Dall R, Hosoda H, et al. Weight loss increases circulating levels of ghrelin in human obesity. Clin Endocrinol 2002;56(2):203–6.
36. Bouret SG. Early life origins of obesity: role of hypothalamic programming. J Ped Gastroenterol Nut 2009;48:S31–8.
37. Adamo MRM, LeRoith D. Insulin and insulin-like growth factor receptors in the nervous system. Mol Neurobiol 1989;3:71–100.
38. Sipols AJ, Baskin DG, Schwartz MW. Effect of intracerebroventricular insulin infusion on diabetic hyperphagia and hypothalamic neuropeptide gene expression. Diabetes 1995;44:147–51.
39. Brennan AM, Mantzoros CS. Drug insight: the role of leptin in human physiology and pathophysiology–emerging clinical applications. Nat Clin Pract Endocrinol Metab 2006;2(6):318–27.
40. Margetic S, Gazzola C, Pegg GG, et al. Leptin: a review of its peripheral actions and interactions. Int J Obes Relat Metab Disord 2002;26(11):1407–33.
41. Tschop M, Smiley DL, Heiman ML. Ghrelin induces adiposity in rodents. Nature 2000;407(6806):908–13.
42. Asakawa A, Inui A, Kaga T, et al. Ghrelin is an appetite-stimulatory signal from stomach with structural resemblance to motilin. Gastroenterology 2001;120(2): 337–45.
43. Inui A. Ghrelin: an orexigenic and somatotrophic signal from the stomach. Nat Rev Neurosci 2001;2(8):551–60.
44. Chen H, Simar D, Morris MJ. Hypothalamic neuroendocrine circuitry is programmed by maternal obesity: interaction with postnatal nutritional environment. PLoS ONE 2009;4(7):e6259.
45. Elias CF, Lee C, Kelly J, et al. Leptin activates hypothalamic CART neurons projecting to the spinal cord. Neuron 1998;21(6):1375–85.
46. Butler AA, Trevaskis JL, Morrison CD. Neuroendocrine control of food intake. In: Bray G, Ryan D, editors. Overweight and the metabolic syndrome: from bench to bedside. Endocrine updates, vol. 26. New York (NY): Springer; 2006. p. 1–10.
47. Heymsfield SB, Greenberg AS, Fujioka K, et al. Recombinant leptin for weight loss in obese and lean adults: a randomized, controlled, dose-escalation trial. JAMA 1999;282(16):1568–75.
48. Neary MT, Batterham RL. Gut hormones: implications for the treatment of obesity. Pharmacol Ther 2009;124(1):44–56.
49. Meier JJ, Nauck MA. Glucagon-like peptide 1(GLP-1) in biology and pathology. Diabetes Metab Res Rev 2005;21(2):91–117.
50. Verdich C, Flint A, Gutzwiller JP, et al. A meta-analysis of the effect of glucagon-like peptide-1 (7-36) amide on ad libitum energy intake in humans. J Clin Endocrinol Metab 2001;86(9):4382–9.
51. le Roux CW, Batterham RL, Aylwin SJB, et al. Attenuated peptide YY release in obese subjects is associated with reduced satiety. Endocrinology 2006;147(1): 3–8.
52. Onaga T, Zabielski R, Kato S. Multiple regulation of peptide YY secretion in the digestive tract. Peptides 2002;23(2):279–90.
53. Feinle-Bisset C, Patterson M, Ghatei MA, et al. Fat digestion is required for suppression of ghrelin and stimulation of peptide YY and pancreatic polypeptide secretion by intraduodenal lipid. Am J Physiol Endocrinol Metab 2005; 289(6):E948–53.
54. Dakin CL, Small CJ, Batterham RL, et al. Peripheral oxyntomodulin reduces food intake and body weight gain in rats. Endocrinology 2004;145(6):2687–95.

55. Wynne K, Park AJ, Small CJ, et al. Oxyntomodulin increases energy expenditure in addition to decreasing energy intake in overweight and obese humans: a randomised controlled trial. Int J Obes 2006;30(12):1729–36.

56. Baggio LL, Huang Q, Brown TJ, et al. Oxyntomodulin and glucagon-like peptide-1 differentially regulate murine food intake and energy expenditure. Gastroenterology 2004;127(2):546–58.

57. Gibbs J, Young RC, Smith GP. Cholecystokinin decreases food intake in rats. J Comp Physiol Psychol 1973;84(3):488–95.

58. Dockray G. Gut endocrine secretions and their relevance to satiety. Curr Opin Pharmacol 2004;4(6):557–60.

59. West DB, Fey D, Woods SC. Cholecystokinin persistently suppresses meal size but not food intake in free-feeding rats. Am J Physiol 1984;246(5 Pt 2):R776–87.

60. Dockray GJ. Peptides of the gut and brain: the cholecystokinins. Proc Nutr Soc 1987;46(1):119–24.

61. Moran TH. Cholecystokinin and satiety: current perspectives. Nutrition 2000; 16(10):858–65.

62. Gurevich-Panigrahi T, Panigrahi S, Wiechec E, et al. Obesity: pathophysiology and clinical management. Curr Med Chem 2009;16(4):506–21.

63. Sarac F, Pehlivan M, Celebi G, et al. Effects of sibutramine on thermogenesis in obese patients assessed via immersion calorimetry. Adv Ther 2006;23(6): 1016–29.

64. Perrio MJ, Wilton LV, Shakir SAW. The safety profiles of orlistat and sibutramine: results of prescription-event monitoring studies in England. Obesity (Silver Spring) 2007;15(11):2712–22.

65. Fich A, Neri M, Camilleri M, et al. Stasis syndromes following gastric surgery: clinical and motility features of 60 symptomatic patients. J Clin Gastroenterol 1990;12(5):505–12.

66. Lakhani SV, Shah HN, Alexander K, et al. Small intestinal bacterial overgrowth and thiamine deficiency after Roux-en-Y gastric bypass surgery in obese patients. Nutr Res 2008;28(5):293–8.

67. German AJ, Day MJ, Ruaux CG, et al. Comparison of direct and indirect tests for small intestinal bacterial overgrowth and antibiotic-responsive diarrhea in dogs. J Vet Intern Med 2003;17(1):33–43 [see comment].

68. Rutgers HC, Batt RM, Elwood CM, et al. Small intestinal bacterial overgrowth in dogs with chronic intestinal disease. J Am Vet Med Assoc 1995;206(2):187–93.

69. Sugerman HJ, Kellum JM, DeMaria EJ. Conversion of proximal to distal gastric bypass for failed gastric bypass for superobesity. J Gastrointest Surg 1997;1(6): 517–24 [discussion: 524–6].

70. Tack J, Arts J, Caenepeel P, et al. Pathophysiology, diagnosis and management of postoperative dumping syndrome. Nat Rev Gastroenterol Hepatol 2009; 6(10):583–90.

71. Halverson JD. Micronutrient deficiencies after gastric bypass for morbid obesity. Am Surg 1986;52(11):594–8.

72. Dowd J. Nutrition management after gastric bypass surgery. Diabetes Spectrum 2005;18(2):82–4.

73. Caruana JA, McCabe MN, Smith AD, et al. Incidence of symptomatic gallstones after gastric bypass: is prophylactic treatment really necessary? Surg Obes Relat Dis 2005;1(6):564–7 [discussion: 567–8].

74. Blachar A, Federle MP, Pealer KM, et al. Gastrointestinal complications of laparoscopic Roux-en-Y gastric bypass surgery: clinical and imaging findings. Radiology 2002;223(3):625–32.

75. Maggard MA, Shugarman LR, Suttorp M, et al. Meta-analysis: surgical treatment of obesity. Ann Intern Med 2005;142(7):547–59.

76. Brolin RE. Bariatric surgery and long-term control of morbid obesity. JAMA 2002;288(22):2793–6.

77. Delin CR, Watts JM, Saebel JL, et al. Eating behavior and the experience of hunger following gastric bypass surgery for morbid obesity. Obes Surg 1997; 7(5):405–13.

78. Morinigo R, Moize V, Musri M, et al. Glucagon-like peptide-1, peptide YY, hunger, and satiety after gastric bypass surgery in morbidly obese subjects. J Clin Endocrinol Metab 2006;91(5):1735–40.

79. Woods SC, Schwartz MW, Baskin DG, et al. Food intake and the regulation of body weight. Annu Rev Psychol 2000;51:255–77.

80. Korner J, Inabnet W, Febres G, et al. Prospective study of gut hormone and metabolic changes after adjustable gastric banding and Roux-en-Y gastric bypass. Int J Obes 2009;33(7):786–95.

81. le Roux CW, Welbourn R, Werling M, et al. Gut hormones as mediators of appetite and weight loss after Roux-en-Y gastric bypass. Ann Surg 2007;246(5): 780–5.

82. Vincent RP, le Roux CW. Changes in gut hormones after bariatric surgery. Clin Endocrinol 2008;69(2):173–9.

83. Dixon AFR, Dixon JB, O'Brien PE. Laparoscopic adjustable gastric banding induces prolonged satiety: a randomized blind crossover study. J Clin Endocrinol Metab 2005;90(2):813–9.

84. Cummings DE, Overduin J, Foster-Schubert KE, et al. Role of the bypassed proximal intestine in the anti-diabetic effects of bariatric surgery. Surg Obes Relat Dis 2007;3(2):109–15.

85. Dixon JB, O'Brien PE, Playfair J, et al. Adjustable gastric banding and conventional therapy for type 2 diabetes: a randomized controlled trial. JAMA 2008; 299(3):316–23.

86. Talley NJ, Quan C, Jones MP, et al. Association of upper and lower gastrointestinal tract symptoms with body mass index in an Australian cohort. Neurogastroenterol Motil 2004;16(4):413–9.

87. Levy RL, Linde JA, Feld KA, et al. The association of gastrointestinal symptoms with weight, diet, and exercise in weight-loss program participants. Clin Gastroenterol Hepatol 2005;3(10):992–6.

88. Nguyen DM, El-Serag HB. The big burden of obesity. Gastrointest Endosc 2009; 70(4):752–7.

89. El-Serag HB, Graham DY, Satia JA, et al. Obesity is an independent risk factor for GERD symptoms and erosive esophagitis. Am J Gastroenterol 2005;100(6): 1243–50.

90. Friedenberg FK, Xanthopoulos M, Foster GD, et al. The association between gastroesophageal reflux disease and obesity. Am J Gastroenterol 2008; 103(8):2111–22.

91. Hampel H, Abraham NS, El-Serag HB. Meta-analysis: obesity and the risk for gastroesophageal reflux disease and its complications. Ann Intern Med 2005; 143(3):199–211.

92. El-Serag H. The association between obesity and GERD: a review of the epidemiological evidence. Dig Dis Sci 2008;53(9):2307–12.

93. Renehan AG, Tyson M, Egger M, et al. Body-mass index and incidence of cancer: a systematic review and meta-analysis of prospective observational studies. Lancet 2008;371(9612):569–78.

94. Corley DA, Kubo A, Zhao W. Abdominal obesity, ethnicity and gastro-oesopha-geal reflux symptoms. Gut 2007;56(6):756–62.
95. Edelstein ZR, Farrow DC, Bronner MP, et al. Central adiposity and risk of Barrett's esophagus. Gastroenterology 2007;133(2):403–11.
96. Corley DA, Kubo A, Levin TR, et al. Abdominal obesity and body mass index as risk factors for Barrett's esophagus. Gastroenterology 2007;133(1):34–41.
97. Cook MB, Greenwood DC, Hardie LJ, et al. A systematic review and meta-anal-ysis of the risk of increasing adiposity on Barrett's esophagus. Am J Gastroen-terol 2008;103(2):292–300.
98. Shaffer EA. Gallstone disease: epidemiology of gallbladder stone disease. Best Pract Res Clin Gastroenterol 2006;20(6):981–96.
99. Li VKM, Pulido N, Fajnwaks P, et al. Predictors of gallstone formation after bari-atric surgery: a multivariate analysis of risk factors comparing gastric bypass, gastric banding, and sleeve gastrectomy. Surg Endosc 2009;23(7):1640–4.
100. Clark JM, Brancati FL, Diehl AM. Nonalcoholic fatty liver disease. Gastroenter-ology 2002;122(6):1649–57.
101. Marceau P, Biron S, Hould FS, et al. Liver pathology and the metabolic syndrome X in severe obesity. J Clin Endocrinol Metab 1999;84(5):1513–7.
102. Diehl AM. Hepatic complications of obesity. Gastroenterol Clin North Am 2005; 34(1):45–61.
103. Halverson JD, Wise L, Wazna MF, et al. Jejunoileal bypass for morbid obesity. A critical appraisal. Am J Med 1978;64(3):461–75.
104. Dhabuwala A, Cannan RJ, Stubbs RS. Improvement in co-morbidities following weight loss from gastric bypass surgery. Obes Surg 2000;10(5):428–35.
105. Wanless IR, Lentz JS. Fatty liver hepatitis (steatohepatitis) and obesity: an autopsy study with analysis of risk factors. Hepatology 1990;12(5):1106–10.
106. Larsson SC, Wolk A. Overweight, obesity and risk of liver cancer: a meta-anal-ysis of cohort studies. Br J Cancer 2007;97(7):1005–8.
107. Ansary Moghaddam A, Wodward M, Huxley R. Obesity and risk of colorectal cancer: a meta-analysis of 31 studies with 70,000 events. Cancer Epidemiol Biomarkers Prev 2007;16:2533–47.
108. Siddiqui A, Pena Sahdala HN, Nazario HE, et al. Obesity is associated with an increased prevalence of advanced adenomatous colon polyps in a male veteran population. Dig Dis Sci 2009;54(7):1560–4.

Gastroesophageal Reflux Disease and Obesity

Girish Anand, MD[a], Philip O. Katz, MD[a,b],*

KEYWORDS

- Gastroesophageal reflux disease • Obesity • Esophagitis
- Lower esophageal sphincter

Gastroesophageal reflux disease (GERD) is a common condition, with multifactorial pathogenesis, affecting up to 40% of the population. Obesity is also common.[1] Obesity and GERD are clearly related, both from a prevalence and causality association. GERD symptoms increase in severity when people gain weight. Obese patients tend to have more severe erosive esophagitis and obesity is a risk factor for the development of Barrett's esophagus and adenocarcinoma of the esophagus. Patients report improvement in GERD when they lose weight and there are several reports suggesting a decrease in GERD symptoms after bariatric surgery. At present, there is little evidence that obesity has any effect on the efficacy of antisecretory therapy, with conflicting data on surgical outcomes. This review attempts to put in perspective the relationship of these two common entities.

DIET, FOOD, AND REFLUX

The major pathophysiologic abnormality in GERD is dysfunction of the lower esophageal sphincter (LES), either manifest as a low resting pressure, or due to a spontaneous decrease in LES pressure due to sphincter shortening in response to gastric distention, a so called transient lower esophageal sphincter relaxation (TLESR). Variability in basal or resting LES pressure and frequency of TLESR makes understanding the effect of food and meal composition on GERD, complex. LES pressure in normals is decreased by fat, which also increases the frequency of TLESR's. This potentially will predispose to increase in GERD symptoms. TLESR frequency is increased by distension of the gastric fundus, so any meal, regardless of its composition will have the potential to promote reflux. It is also clear that there is a relationship between

[a] Division of Gastroenterology, Albert Einstein Medical Center, 5401 Old York Road, Klein Professional Building, Suite 363, Philadelphia, PA 19141, USA
[b] Thomas Jefferson University, Philadelphia, PA, USA
* Corresponding author. Division of Gastroenterology, Albert Einstein Medical Center, 5401 Old York Road, Klein Professional Building, Suite 363, Philadelphia, PA 19141.
E-mail address: 19141.katzp@einstein.edu (P.O. Katz).

Gastroenterol Clin N Am 39 (2010) 39–46
doi:10.1016/j.gtc.2009.12.002
0889-8553/10/$ – see front matter © 2010 Elsevier Inc. All rights reserved.

the speed at which one eats and postprandial reflux. A meal eaten in less than 5 minutes results in more postprandial reflux than a meals eaten over 30 minutes.[2]

There are few studies on LES function in the obese. The limited data suggests that basal pressure in the morbidly obese is similar to those of ideal body weight.[3] Hiatal hernia is more often seen in patients with obesity and the authors' clinical impression is that they tend to be larger in the obese.[4,5] The relationship between obesity and esophageal motility function, notably TLESR, has recently been studied in subjects with GERD and hiatus hernia. Obesity is associated with increased TLESR, postprandial gastroesophageal reflux (GER), and esophageal acid exposure. The frequency of TLESR is correlated with increased body mass index (BMI) and waist circumference.[6] The pressure profile within and across the gastroesophageal junction in the obese is altered in a way that increases GER. During inspiration, increased intragastric pressure and the gastroesophageal pressure gradient are correlated with increased BMI. The changes noted above are more strongly correlated with waist circumference. The speculation is that waist circumference is the mediator of the obesity effect on GERD. Obesity is associated with increased axial separation between the LES and the extrinsic crural diaphragm, indicating anatomic disruption of the esophageal junction, which likely contributes in the development of hiatal hernia. These findings offer a physiologic explanation for the effect of obesity on GERD.[7] A rise in intra-abdominal pressure in obesity may cause the cephalad movement of a hiatus hernia, predisposing to reflux.[8] Gastric volume and gastric emptying are normal in the limited studies in obese subjects.[9] One study demonstrated higher maximal gastric acid response to gastrin stimulation[10]—but gastric acid production is probably normal.[11] There is an association between obesity and intraesophageal acid exposure, likely mediated by waist circumference.[12] Acid sensitivity may be increased in the obese compared with those of normal body weight.[13] To summarize these studies: obese subjects are more likely to have a hiatal hernia, increased intragastric pressure, and an augmented gastroesophageal pressure gradient—providing the ideal situation for reflux. Abdominal obesity, specifically a greater waist circumference, is likely the mediator of the effect of increased body weight on gastric pressure.[7] Finally, gastric emptying is delayed after large meals and after high-calorie meals. Accordingly, a large, high-fat meal would predispose to TLESR and a greater risk for reflux **(Table 1)**.[14]

SYMPTOMS

Studies investigating the association of GERD symptoms and obesity are conflicting. A large population study from Sweden did not demonstrate a relationship between

Table 1 Factors predisposing obese patients to GERD	
Mechanical	Increased intra-gastric pressure Increased gastroesophageal pressure gradient Increased in hiatal hernia Increased esophageal acid sensitivity
Physiological	Increased bile & pepsin composition of gastric content and increased outputs of bile and pancreatic secretions Higher maximal gastric acid response to graded intravenous pentagastrin Lack of suppression of basal gastric acid secretion after intravenous secretin Reduced cholecystokinin-stimulated pancreatic enzyme secretion, bile acid emptying, and gastrin release

BMI and symptoms.[15] A meta-analysis in the United States found a positive association between the presence of GERD and increasing BMI.[16] Other large-scale studies have shown that GERD is common in the general population and especially so among the overweight. A strong positive association between BMI and symptoms of GERD was found in a recent cross-sectional study in a large cohort of women. An increase in BMI of more than 3.5 kg/m^2, as compared with no weight changes, was associated with an increased risk of frequency of GERD symptoms.[17] A BMI over 30 kg/m^2 was associated with a three-fold increase in the odds of having frequent reflux symptoms.[18] Weight gain increased risk of symptoms of GERD and weight loss decreased risk.[17] A dose-response relationship between BMI and the risk of reporting symptoms of GERD among both men and women was seen in a recent meta-analysis. A BMI between 25 and 29 kg/m^2 and a BMI greater than 30 kg/m^2 were associated with an increased risk for GERD symptoms—odds ratios of 1.43 and 1.94 respectively ($P<.001$).[19] There was a higher hospitalization rate for reflux codes in patients with an elevated BMI compared with normal-weight controls in a recent cross-sectional study.[20] An increase in BMI is associated with an incremental increase in the risk of developing GERD symptoms.[21] The difference was not as dramatic, but there was a significant statistical trend toward more severe symptoms in the obese—particularly in women—compared with the ideal body weight population.[22,23]

The Progression of Gastroesophageal Reflux Disease (ProGERD) study (N = 6215), found that a higher BMI was associated with more frequent and more severe heartburn, regurgitation, and erosive esophagitis. The findings were more pronounced for regurgitation than heartburn. Obese women had an increased risk of severe esophagitis compared with women with normal weight (odds ratio 2.51, 95%CI 1.53–4.12).[24] There was, however, no difference evident in men.

Contradictory results have been seen in evaluating esophageal acid exposure in obesity. A small study found 64% of patients in a bariatric surgery program had abnormal ambulatory 24-hour esophageal acid exposure, higher than asymptomatic volunteers ($P = .04$).[25] In addition, heartburn, acid regurgitation, dysphagia, and asthma were more prevalent in the bariatric surgery patients than in the general population. Fifty consecutive obese patients referred for bariatric surgery had 24-hour ambulatory pH and endoscopy findings similar to the general population.[26] An additional study found a BMI greater than 30 kg/m^2 to be associated with a significant increase in the number of reflux episodes, reflux episodes of less than 5 minutes, and total and percent time with pH less than 4, especially in the postprandial period. Waist circumference was associated with esophageal acid exposure, but was not as significant or consistent as BMI.[27] An independent association between increasing abdominal diameter (independent of BMI) and reflux-type symptoms was seen in whites, but not in blacks or Asians. Perhaps increased obesity may disproportionately increase GERD-type symptoms in whites and in males.[28] Overall, the weight of the epidemiologic evidence supports an association between GERD and obesity.

COMPLICATIONS

A recent meta-analysis showed a statistically significant increase in the risk for GERD symptoms, erosive esophagitis, esophageal adenocarcinoma, and a progressive increase with increasing weight. A BMI greater than 25 kg/m^2 had an odds ratio of 1.76 for erosive esophagitis and 2.02 for esophageal adenocarcinoma, compared with patients with normal weight ($P<.001$).[19] Four prospective multicenter, randomized, double blind trials comparing esomeprazole and other proton pump inhibitors in patients with *Helicobacter pylori*-negative serology found weak but statistically significant risk for Los Angeles grades C and D erosive esophagitis, but not grades A and B, in the obese.[29] Similar results have been published regarding the Chinese.[30] The ProGERD study identified several independent risk factors for erosive esophagitis including BMI. As BMI rose, the odds for higher degrees of erosive esophagitis increased.[31] Though other studies fail to show an increase in erosive esophagitis in obese patients with GERD, the balance of the evidence seems to indicate a relationship.

A case-control study evaluated cases with Barrett's esophagus and 2 control groups: normal-weight patients and patients with GERD but without Barrett's esophagus. Abdominal diameter was an independent risk factor for Barrett's esophagus. There was no association between Barrett's esophagus and BMI.[32]

There is a well-documented association between BMI and carcinoma of the esophagus and gastric cardia.[33–35] This is perhaps the most concerning and distressing link between obesity and its effect on the natural history and severity of GERD.

WEIGHT LOSS

The majority of studies examining the effect of nonsurgical weight loss on GERD show no effect or symptoms, endoscopic findings, or pH monitoring.[36,37] A cross-sectional study demonstrated a nearly 40% reduction in the risk of frequent GERD symptoms in women with a decrease in BMI of more than 3.5 kg/m^2 compared with those without a change in BMI (odds ratio 0.64).[17] Another study (N = 34) of subjects with a BMI greater than 23 kg/m^2 found that GERD symptoms improved by 75% from baseline with a mean weight loss of 4 kg. There was a direct correlation between weight loss and symptom score.[38] Improvement in reflux symptoms has been suggested after bariatric procedures—particularly the Roux-en-Y gastric bypass (RYGB), which has an antireflux component.[39–41] There is near-complete cessation of acid production because of a small proximal gastric cardia pouch and complete diversion of duodenal contents, making the RYGB, in theory, the optimal antireflux procedure. There are no prospective studies examining the relationship of obesity and the outcome of traditional medical therapy in GERD or on whether obesity affects pharmacodynamics or pharmacokinetics of proton pump inhibitors. A retrospective review of a large database found similar healing rates for erosive esophagitis in overweight compared with normal patients, suggesting body weight did not affect healing of esophagitis with proton pump inhibitors.[42]

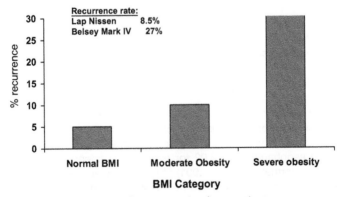

Fig. 1. Higher failure rate for antireflux surgery in obese patients.

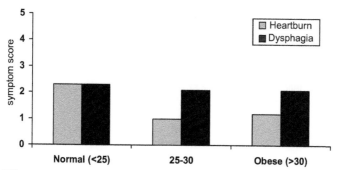

Fig. 2. No difference in surgical outcome regardless of preoperative weight.

TREATMENT: APPROACH TO THE PATIENT

As there are no data specifically related to treatment of GERD in the obese, the authors approach obese patients with GERD in the same way as patients with GERD who are ideal body weight. We discuss lifestyle modifications, start therapy with a proton pump inhibitor once daily before breakfast for 4 to 8 weeks, and adjust therapy based on response.

There are no studies of endoscopic therapies (endoluminal gastric plication, radiofrequency energy ablation) in patients with BMI greater than 30 or 35 kg/m^2 because these patients were excluded from the trials. Hence, there is no way of knowing what the success of endoscopic therapy would be if it were available.

Antireflux surgery is a maintenance option for patients with GERD. Current data in overweight patients suggest that fundoplication and RYGB can be effective in long-term surgical treatment of GERD. However, fundoplication has lower perioperative risks and excellent outcomes in overweight patients (BMI 25–29.9 kg/m^2) with GERD who do not have serious weight-related morbidity. The authors suggest that patients with class II obesity (BMI 35–39.9 kg/m^2)—especially those with weight-related comorbidities or class III obesity (BMI>40 kg/m^2) regardless of other comorbidities—consider a bariatric procedure. Several bariatric procedures such as RYGB and gastric banding have been reported to reduce symptoms and esophageal acid exposure. Studies evaluating the results of fundoplication in the obese are conflicting. A high rate of recurrence (31%) was seen in patients with BMI greater than 30 kg/m^2 compared with 8% in patients with BMI between 25 and 29.9 kg/m^2, and only 4.5% in patients with BMIs less than 25 kg/m^2 (**Fig. 1**).[43] Another study found no difference in symptom scores after antireflux surgery in those of normal body weight compared with the obese (**Fig. 2**).[44] In a multivariate analysis, obesity was not associated with worse outcomes for fundoplication.[45] A review of 505 patients found no association between BMI and complications or anatomic failure.[46]

Patients with obesity and GERD should be made aware of the multiple surgical and nonsurgical GERD options if they are considering surgical treatment specifically targeting GERD therapy.

SUMMARY

Though direct cause and effect cannot be documented, the majority of the evidence suggests a direct relationship between obesity and GERD. Weight loss should be pursued with expectation that symptoms will improve. However, it is difficult to predict what degree of weight loss is required to alter the pressure profile across the gastroesophageal junction and improve other mechanical factors. Weight loss has beneficial heath effects and this should supersede GERD as the primary reason to lose weight. Evaluation and treatment of the obese patient with GERD should follow the same principles as in a patient with normal body weight. Though the frequency of complications may be higher, no definitive study is available to suggest deviating from current guidelines. Prospective studies directed at the obese patient are clearly needed to determine if different approaches are required.

REFERENCES

1. Flegal KM, Carroll MD, Ogden CL, et al. Prevalence and trends in obesity among US adults, 1999–2000. JAMA 2002;288:1723–7.
2. Wildi SM, Tutuian R, Castell DO. The influence of rapid food intake on postprandial reflux: studies in healthy volunteers. Am J Gastroenterol 2004;99:1645–51.
3. O'Brien TF Jr. Lower esophageal sphincter pressure (LESP) and esophageal function in obese humans. J Clin Gastroenterol 1980;2:145–8.
4. Stene-Larsen G, Weberg R, Froyshov Larsen I, et al. Relationship of overweight to hiatus hernia and reflux oesophagitis. Scand J Gastroenterol 1988;23:427–32.
5. Wilson LJ, Ma W, Hirschowtiz BI. Association of obesity with hiatal hernia and esophagitis. Am J Gastroenterol 1999;94:2840–4.
6. Wu JC, Mui LM, Cheung CM, et al. Obesity is associated with increased transient lower esophageal sphincter relaxation. Gastroenterology 2007;132(3):883–9.
7. Pandolfino JE, El-Serag HB, Zhang Q, et al. Obesity: a challenge to esophagogastric junction integrity. Gastroenterology 2006;130(3):639–49.
8. Sugerman HJ, DeMaria EJ, Felton WL III, et al. Increased intra-abdominal pressure and cardiac filling pressures in obesity-associated pseudotumor cerebri. Neurology 1997;49:507–11.
9. Wisen O, Johansson C. Gastrointestinal function in obesity: motility, secretion, and absorption following a liquid test meal. Meta 1992;41:390–5.
10. Wisen O, Rossner S, Johansson C. Gastric secretion in massive obesity. Evidence of abnormal response to vagal stimulation. Dig Dis Sci 1987;32:968–72.
11. Harter RL, Kelly WB, Kramer MG, et al. A comparison of the volume and pH of gastric contents of obese and lean surgical patients. Anesth Analg 1998;86:147–52.
12. Crowell MD, Hansel BA, Dionisio P, et al. Obesity is associated with increased 48-h esophageal acid exposure in patients with symptomatic gastroesophageal reflux. Am J Gastroenterol 2009;104(3):553–9.
13. Mercer CD, Wren SF, DaCosta LR, et al. Lower esophageal sphincter pressure and gastroesophageal pressure gradients in excessively obese patients. J Med 1987;18:135–46.
14. Kendrick ML, Houghton SG. Gastroesophageal reflux disease in obese patients: the role of obesity in management. Dis Esophagus 2006;19(2):57–63.
15. Lagergren J, Bergstrom R, Nyren O. No relation between body mass and gastroesophageal reflux symptoms in a Swedish population based study. Gut 2000;47:26–9.
16. Corley DA, Kubo A. Body mass index and gastroesophageal reflux disease: a systematic review and meta-analysis. Am J Gastroenterol 2006;101(11):2619–28.
17. Jacobson BC, Somers SC, Fuchs CS, et al. Body-mass index and symptoms of gastroesophageal reflux in women. N Engl J Med 2006;354(22):2340–8.

18. Locke GR, Talley NJ, Fett SL, et al. Risk factors associated with symptoms of gastroesophageal reflux. Am J Med 1999;106:642–9.
19. Hampel H, Abraham NS, El-Serag HB. Meta-analysis: obesity and the risk for gastroesophageal reflux disease and its complications. Ann Intern Med 2005; 143(3):199–211.
20. Ruhl CE, Everhart JE. Overweight, but not high dietary fat intake, increases risk of gastroesophageal reflux disease hospitalization: The NHANES I Epidemiologic follow up study. First National Health and Nutrition Examination Survey. Ann Epidemiol 1999;9:424–35.
21. Nandurkar S, Locke GR 3rd, Fett S, et al. Relationship between body mass index, diet, exercise and gastro-oesophageal reflux symptoms in a community. Aliment Pharmacol Ther 2004;20(5):497–505.
22. Murray L, Johnston B, Lane A, et al. Relationship between body mass and gastro-oesophageal reflux symptoms: the Bristol Helicobacter project. Int J Epidemiol 2003;32:645–50.
23. Nilsson M, Johnsen R, Ye W, et al. Obesity and estrogen as risk factors for gastro-esophageal reflux symptoms. JAMA 2003;290:66–72.
24. Nocon M, Labenz J, Jaspersen D, et al. Association of body mass index with heartburn, regurgitation, and esophagitis: results of the progression of gastro-esophageal reflux disease study. J Gastroenterol Hepatol 2007;22(11):1728–31.
25. Talley NJ, Howell S, Poulton R. Obesity and chronic gastrointestinal tract symptoms in young adults: a birth cohort study. Am J Gastroenterol 2004;99: 1807–14.
26. Lundell L, Ruth M, Sandberg N, et al. Does massive obesity promote abnormal gastroesophageal reflux? Dig Dis Sci 1995;40:1632–5.
27. El-Serag HB, Ergun GA, Pandolfino J, et al. Obesity increases esophageal acid exposure. Gut 2007;56(6):749–55.
28. Corley DA, Kubo A, Zhao W. Abdominal obesity, ethnicity, and gastroesophageal reflux symptoms. Gut 2007;56(6):756–62.
29. El-Serag HB, Johanson JF. Risk factors for the severity of erosive esophagitis in Helicobacter pylori-negative patients with gastroesophageal reflux disease. Scand J Gastroenterol 2002;37(8):899–904.
30. Chang CS, Poon SK, Lien HC, et al. The incidence of reflux esophagitis among the Chinese. Am J Gastroenterol 1997;92:668–71.
31. Labenz J, Jasperson D, Kulig M, et al. Risk factors for erosive esophagitis: a multi-variate analysis based on the ProGERD study initiative. Am J Gastroenterol 2004; 99:1652–6.
32. Corley DA, Kubo A, Levin TR, et al. Abdominal obesity and body mass index as risk factors for Barrett's esophagus. Gastroenterology 2007;133(1):34–41.
33. Lagergren J, Bergstrom R, Nyren O. Association between body mass and adeno-carcinoma of the esophagus and gastric cardia. Ann Intern Med 1999;130: 883–90.
34. Engel LS, Chow WH, Vaughan TL, et al. Population attributable risks of esopha-geal and gastric cancers. J Natl Cancer Inst 2003;95:1404–13.
35. Pohl H, Robertson D. Obesity—should we worry about esophageal adenocarci-noma? [abstract 87]. Am J Gastroenterol 2004;99(10):S29.
36. Mathus-Vliegen EM, van Weeren M, Van Eerten PV. LOS function and obesity: the impact of untreated obesity, weight loss, and chronic gastric balloon distension. Digestion 2003;68:161–8.
37. Kjellin A, Ramel S, Rossner S, et al. Gastroesophageal reflux in obese patients is not reduced by weight reduction. Scand J Gastroenterol 1996;31:1047–51.

38. Fraser-Moodie CA, Norton B, Gornall C, et al. Weight loss has an independent beneficial effect on symptoms of gastro-oesophageal reflux in patients who are overweight. Scand J Gastroenterol 1999;4:337–40.

39. Jones KB Jr, Allen TV, Manas KJ, et al. Roux-Y Gastric bypass: an effective anti-reflux procedure. Obes Surg 1991;1(3):295–8.

40. Jones KB Jr. Roux-en-Y gastric bypass: an effective antireflux procedure in the less than morbidly obese. Obes Surg 1998;8(1):35–8.

41. Smith SC, Edwards CB, Goodman GN. Symptomatic and clinical improvement in morbidly obese patients with gastroesophageal reflux disease following Roux-en-Y gastric bypass. Obes Surg 1997;7(6):479–84.

42. Vakil N, Sharma P, Monyak JT, et al. Is obesity the cause of reduced healing rates in advanced grades of erosive esophagitis (EE)? [abstract]. Am J Gastroenterol 2007;102(S2):S445.

43. Perez AR, Moncure AC, Rattner DW. Obesity adversely affects the outcome of antireflux operations. Surg Endosc 2002;15:986–9.

44. Fraser J, Watson DI, O'Boyle CJ, et al. Obesity and its effect on outcome of laparoscopic Nissen fundoplication. Dis Esophagus 2001;14:50–3.

45. Peters JH, DeMeester TR, Oberg S, et al. Multivariate analysis of factors predicting outcome after laparoscopic Nissen fundoplication. J Gastrointest Surg 1999; 3(3):292–300.

46. Winslow ER, Frisella MM, Soper NJ, et al. Obesity does not adversely affect the outcome of laparoscopic antireflux surgery (LARS). Surg Endosc 2003;17(12): 2003–11.

Colonic Complications of Obesity

Carol A. Burke, MD

KEYWORDS

- Colorectal neoplasia • Colon cancer
- Colorectal adenoma • Obesity

Cancer and cardiovascular disease are the leading causes of death in American men and women. Obesity, which is due, in part, to excess food intake coupled with physical inactivity, increases the risk of both diseases. The physiologic basis for the detrimental effects of obesity on the colon is not understood but the complex interactions between adipocytokines, colonocytes and diet are being investigated. Central (abdominal distribution) but more specifically, visceral adipose tissue (VAT), is suggested to be fundamental for the development of the obesity-related metabolic changes leading to systemic disease. The most well-studied effect of obesity is its association with colorectal neoplasia; lesser known effects include a heightened risk of complications of diverticulosis, inadequate bowel preparation, and a poorer postoperative outcome after colon surgery.

It has been recognized from numerous epidemiologic studies that a relationship exists between body mass index (BMI) and disease, including mortality. In 1 cohort study of more than 1 million American adults, the relationship between BMI and death was found to be curvilinear. The nadir of mortality was found at a BMI of 23.5 to 24.9 kg/m^2 in men and 22.0 to 23.4 kg/m^2 in women. The relative risk (RR) of death at both extremes, at a BMI of less than 18.5 kg/m^2 and equal to or greater than 40 kg/m^2, was approximately 80% higher than subjects in the range at the nadir.[1] In the cohort, BMI was also associated with death from cancer. The risk increased linearly above the nadir, throughout the range of BMI in the overweight (>25 kg/m^2) and obese ($\geq$30 kg/m^2) range, without an observed risk for leaner individuals. Data from a European cohort of more than 350,000 individuals confirmed the parabolic nature between BMI and mortality. The lowest risks of death were at a BMI of 25.3 kg/m^2 for men and 24.3 kg/m^2 for women.[2] Subjects in this cohort had additional measures of obesity recorded. Their waist was measured at its narrowest circumference of the torso or at the midpoint between the lower ribs and iliac crest. Hip circumference was measured at the largest extension of the hips over the buttocks. Both waist circumference (WC) and

Department of Gastroenterology and Hepatology, Center for Colon Polyp and Cancer Prevention, Digestive Disease Institute, Cleveland Clinic, Desk A30, 9500 Euclid Avenue, Cleveland, OH 44195, USA
E-mail address: Burkec1@ccf.org

Gastroenterol Clin N Am 39 (2010) 47–55
doi:10.1016/j.gtc.2009.12.005
0889-8553/10/$ – see front matter © 2010 Elsevier Inc. All rights reserved.

waist-to-hip ratio (WHR) were independent predictors for death. RRs of death among men and women in the highest quintile of WC were 2.05 (95% CI 1.80–2.33) and 1.78 (95% CI 1.56–2.04) and in the highest quintile of WHR the RRs were 1.68 (95% CI 1.53–1.84) and 1.51(95% CI 1.37–1.66), respectively.

Variable risk estimates for the association of obesity with colonic disease have been obtained and reflect the effect of gender and differences in the anthropometric measures used to determine adiposity. BMI is the most common measure of obesity and is derived from the Quetelet index. BMI is an estimation of general adiposity that compares a person's weight and height (**Table 1**). BMI is determined by weight in kilograms divided by the square of height in meters.[3] The World Health Organization (WHO) defines overweight as a BMI of 25 to 29.9 kg/m^2 and obese as a BMI equal to or greater than 30 kg/m^2.

BMI cannot discriminate excess in body fat from increment in lean mass or fat distribution. Because the location of fat distribution seems to be important in determining risk of disease, complementary anthropometric methods have been developed. WC and WHR are surrogate markers of VAT. VAT is believed to be the metabolically active organ responsible for the production of multiple humoral factors and neuronal signaling pathways. Adipocytes produce and secrete cytokines such as leptin, adiponectin, tumor necrosis factor (TNFα), fatty acids, and growth factors, which have effects on glucose and lipid metabolism, cell proliferation, inflammation, oxidative stress, and energy homeostasis.

OBESITY AND COLORECTAL NEOPLASIA
Pathophysiology

It has long been recognized that there is a strong environmental component to colorectal cancer. Dietary and other modifiable risk factors are estimated to account for up to 90% of colorectal cancers.[4] Epidemiologic studies have confirmed that a western lifestyle including physical inactivity and high dietary fat and energy intake beyond expenditure, both of which lead to obesity, are important risk factors. The relationship between obesity and colon cancer risk is well studied, however the specific mechanistic pathways that lead to carcinogenesis are not conclusive.[5] The association between the metabolic syndrome and colorectal cancer mortality and type 2 diabetes mellitus with colorectal cancer risk lend support to obesity-induced insulin resistance and hyperinsulinemia as a core pathway. Hyperinsulinemia results in a decrease in IGF-binding protein (IGFBP) and high levels of circulating insulin-like growth factor I

Table 1 Measures of obesity			
	Normal	**Overweight**	**Obese**
BMI	<25	25–29.9	≥30
Waist circumference			
Men	<102 cm or <40 in		
Women	<88 cm or <35 in		
Waist/hip ratio			
Men	1.0		
Women	0.85		

BMI = (weight in kg divided by height in m^2) or ([weight in pounds divided by height in inches^2] × 703).

(IGF-I). Activation of IGF receptors on colonocytes inhibit apoptosis, enhance epithelial cell proliferation and is associated with the development, progression, and metastatic potential of colon cancer. TNF-α, constitutively expressed in adipocytes, attenuates insulin signaling and causes insulin resistance by various mechanisms including inhibition of tyrosine phosphorylation, suppression of cytokine signaling protein 3 synthesis, and stimulation of adipocyte lipolysis leading to hypertriglyceridemia. In addition, obesity is associated with abnormalities in the bioavailability of plasma androgens and estrogens and increases levels of circulating sex hormones as a result of enhanced IGF-1 activity in the liver inhibiting hepatic sex hormone-binding globulin synthesis. Studies in male aromatase knockout mice (ArKO) have shown that a lack of estrogen results in the development of a metabolic syndrome characterized by excess adiposity, hepatic steatosis, and insulin resistance.[6] The increase in androgen to estrogen ratio promotes visceral fat accumulation in the rodent model and leads to death of dopaminergic neurons in the hypothalamic acuate nucleus, which is pivotal to regulation of energy. These effects may account for the heightened risk of colorectal cancer observed in men and premenopausal women compared with postmenopausal women especially if they also take hormone replacement therapy (HRT). Leptin, a cytokine-like peptide, is produced in adipose tissue. It is involved in energy balance, regulation of food intake, and nutrient absorption in enterocytes. Leptin targets the ObRb receptor on colonocytes, leading to expression of transcription factors, cell proliferation, production of proinflammatory cytokines, and oxidative stress. Elevated levels of leptin have been associated with colon cancer although the association is inconsistent. Recent work demonstrates that leptin induces IGF-mediated pathway gene expression in colonocytes with an APC mutation suggesting a potential link between leptin and the increased risk of colon cancer associated with obesity.[7] Leptin triggers an inflammatory response in tumor tissue through direct stimulation of colonocytes, inducing recruitment of cytotoxic T cells into the tumor microenvironment.[8] This tumoral immune response, may be associated with the better prognosis associated with over expression of leptin receptor in patients with colon cancer.[9]

Epidemiologic and randomized controlled trials have shown an inverse association between the risk of colorectal neoplasia and plasma concentrations or intake of calcium and/or vitamin D. Preliminary work on calcium intake, obesity, and insulin resistance in a cross-sectional study found that mean calcium intake was lower in obese adolescents than those of normal weight.[10] Calcium intake was inversely associated with body trunk fat, insulin, and the homeostasis model assessment of insulin resistance (HOMA-IR) in the obese group. Girls in the highest quartile of calcium intake had decreased adiposity and insulin resistance. Greater adiposity has also been associated with lower blood levels of vitamin D and 25-hydroxyvitamin D. In a cross-sectional study of 381 healthy men and women from a randomized trial of calcium and vitamin D supplementation to prevent bone loss, individuals with the highest percentage body fat (>40%) had 20% lower 25-hydroxyvitamin D concentrations than those in the lowest quartile (<28% fat).[11] This study suggests that vitamin D is sequestered in fat tissue, reducing its entry into the circulation and thus may be a factor in the obesity-related risk of neoplasia.

Evidence of an Association Between Obesity and Colorectal Cancer

The positive association between BMI and colon cancer risk has been well studied although some inconsistencies exist, in particular for women. In the NIH-AARP Diet and Health Study on 307,708 men and 209,436 women followed for 4.5 years, BMI showed a strong linear correlation with colon, but not rectal, cancer risk in men and women.[12] The association was seen in younger (50–66 years) but not older (67–71 years) women and was not modified by HRT. The National Health and Nutrition Examination Survey (NHANES) epidemiologic follow-up study of 13,420 individuals in the United States followed up for approximately 15 years showed that baseline BMI in the overweight and obese range is associated with the development of colon cancer in men and women.[13] The hazards ratio were similar for men and women, 2.47 (95% CI 1.14–5.32), 3.72 (95% CI 1.68–8.22), and 2.79 (95% CI 1.22–6.35) for a BMI of 26 to 27.9 kg/m^2, 28 to 29.9 kg/m^2, and 30 kg/m^2 or more, respectively, compared with those with a BMI less than 22 kg/m^2. Subscapular skin fold thickness (which may reflect greater central adiposity), but not triceps skin fold thickness, was associated with colon cancer incidence in men but not women, suggesting that the distribution of adiposity affects the RR in a gender-specific way. To examine the independent effects of the distribution of adiposity on colon cancer risk, follow-up data on 3802 individuals in the Framingham cohort with BMI and WC measures at 2 age periods was analyzed.[14] A BMI of 30 kg/m^2 or more was associated with an increased risk of colon cancer in those aged 30 to 54 years (RR 1.5, 95% CI 0.92–2.5); the RR in those 55–79 years was 2.4 (95% CI 1.5–3.9). The BMI effect was stronger in men than women and for proximal colon cancer. These risks diminished when WC was added to the model. Men and women with a large WC had a 70% increased risk of colon cancer and those with an extra large WC had a 90% increased risk. This effect was not attenuated by BMI suggesting that body fat distribution is an independent risk factor for colon cancer, proximal and distal, in these subjects. Sedentary men and women in the highest WC category had the greatest risk RR of 3.0 (95% CI 1.0–9.1) and 4.4 (95% CI 1.5–12.9), respectively.

The European Prospective Investigation into Cancer and Nutrition (EPIC) examined the association between different anthropometric features and risk of colon and rectal cancer in nearly 370,000 European men and women followed for 6 years.[15] No anthropometric measure was related to rectal cancer risk. A 55% increased risk of colon cancer was observed in men in the highest versus lowest quintiles of BMI but a similar association was not evident in women. WC and WHR were associated with a nearly 50% increased RR of colon cancer in men and women. The association of WC and WHR and colon cancer risk observed among postmenopausal women was ameliorated in those who used HRT.

Two recent meta-analyses have estimated the strength of the association between measures of adiposity and colorectal cancer in men and women.[16,17] In the first publication, the estimated RR of colorectal cancer was 1.19 (95% CI 1.11–1.29) comparing BMI of 30 kg/m^2 or more with BMI less than 25 kg/m^2 and 1.45 (95% CI 1.31–1.61) comparing highest to lowest level of WC. There was a stronger association in men 1.41 (95% CI 1.30–1.54) than women 1.08 (95% CI 0.98–1.18). For every 2 kg/m^2 increase in BMI the risk of developing colorectal cancer increases 7%. Every 2 cm increase in WC is associated with a 4% increased risk of colorectal cancer. The risk was greatest for colon, rather than rectal, cancer and was 30% higher in obese men compared with obese women. In the second analysis, the risks of BMI, WC, and WHR on colorectal cancer were assessed. For each 5-unit increase in BMI, the risk of colon cancer increased in men by 30% (95% CI 1.25–1.35) and in women by 12% (95% CI 1.07–1.18). BMI was associated with rectal cancer in men but not women. Colon cancer risk increased with every 10 cm increase in WC in men by 33% (95% CI 1.19–1.49) and by 16% (95% CI 1.09–1.23) in women, and with increasing WHR per 0.1 unit in men by 1.43 (95% CI 1.19–1.71) and women by 1.20 (95% CI 1.08–1.33).

Although the association between obesity and colorectal cancer seems irrefutable, there is evidence that the association of BMI, percent body fat, and WC on digestive system mortality can be attenuated by higher levels of muscular strength.[18] Overall and site-specific cancer death rates/100,000 person years decreased across incremental thirds of muscular strength in 8677 men. Furthermore, the association between obesity and cancer mortality did not persist after adjusting for muscular strength. The mechanisms that may explain the lower risk of cancer mortality seen in men with higher levels of muscular strength may be through enhancement of insulin sensitivity by physical activity and increased glucose uptake by skeletal muscle.

Evidence of an Association Between Obesity and Adenomas

In addition to the positive association between increasing adiposity and the risk of colorectal cancer, several cross-sectional or case-control studies have also shown a moderately increased risk of obesity for an increased prevalence of colorectal adenomas. Determinants of insulin secretion and insulin-like growth factors have been directly associated with risk for colorectal cancer but few studies have looked at the factors in relation to colorectal adenomas. The Nurses Health Study identified 380 cases with distal colorectal adenomas diagnosed between 1989 and 1998 and 380 controls among nondiabetic women in the cohort of 32,826 women.[19] Individuals in the highest quartile of C-peptide concentrations had the highest risk of adenoma 1.63 (95% CI 1.01–2.66) compared with the bottom quartile. This suggests that hyperinsulinemia may play a role in the development of adenomas. A cohort study on nearly 8000 average-risk Japanese with a mean age of 47.5 years analyzed the effect of being overweight and obese by BMI on the prevalence of colorectal neoplasia at baseline colonoscopy, and incidence of neoplasia in 2568 of the subjects on follow-up colonoscopy 1 year later.[20] Not surprisingly, the prevalence of adenoma at baseline colonoscopy increased proportionally from 15.5%, 20.6%, 22.7% to 24.2% according to quartile of baseline BMI in kg/m^2 (<21.35, ≥21.35 to <23.199, ≥23.199 to <25.156, ≥25.156). The prevalence of multiple adenomas increased in subjects according to the BMI, but no association with large adenomas or adenomas with high-grade dysplasia was noted. The incidence of adenoma on follow-up examination increased proportionally with BMI from 12.9%, 15.7%, 18.3% to 19%. The incidence rates were lowest (9.3%), in subjects who experienced a weight reduction, 16.2% in those with a weight gain, and 17.1% in those with no change in weight (P = .01 reduction vs no reduction groups).

The positive association between obesity, weight gain, and adenoma risk was confirmed in 600 subjects who underwent colonoscopy as part of a prospective multiethnic cohort study called the Insulin Resistance Atherosclerosis Study (IRAS).[21] Obesity, as determined by BMI at the time of colonoscopy, was associated with 2.16 (95% CI 1.13–4.14) risk of adenoma and was stronger in women 4.42 (95% CI 1.53–12.78) than in men 1.26 (95% CI 0.52–3.07). The risk of adenoma increased among participants who gained weight (>4 pounds) in the previous 5 years 2.30 (95% CI 1.25–4.22) and 10 years 2.12 (95% CI 1.25–3.62) compared with those who maintained their weight over the same period. A trend toward a protective benefit was noted in individuals who had a weight loss in the previous 10 years (odds ratio [OR] 0.38, 95% CI 0.13–1.11), but not those who reported a weight loss in the previous 5 years. In this study, the strongest associations with adenoma risk were observed when obesity was measured at the time of colonoscopy, suggesting that obesity may be a promoting factor in the growth of colorectal adenomas.

The Black Women's Health Study followed 33,403 women older than 29 years to determine the risk of adenoma in African American women.[22] The incidence rate ratio

(IRR) comparing women with a current BMI of 35 kg/m^2 or more to less than 25 kg/m^2 was 1.35 (95% CI 1.12–1.62). The IRR, comparing the highest (≥0.87) to lowest (<0.71) quintiles of WHR was 1.26 (95% CI 1.04–1.54). The amount of weight gained since the age of 18 years was significantly associated with the risk of adenoma. Women gaining between 5 and 14 kg of weight had a risk of 1.34 (95% CI 0.99–1.51), those gaining 15–29 kg had a risk of 1.59 (95% CI 1.17–2.15), and those gaining 30 kg or more had a risk of 2.01 (95% CI 1.29–3.13).

Pooled data from 2465 individuals participating in 2 prospective randomized trials comparing the effect of a high versus low fiber diet and the effect of ursodeoxycholic acid on adenoma recurrence were used to assess the association between BMI and WC on adenoma recurrence.[23] BMI was categorized as normal, overweight, or obese and WC (in inches) as small, medium, large, and extra large. Follow-up colonoscopy was done at a mean of 3.1 years after the clearing colonoscopy. The risk of recurrent advanced adenomas was increased in overweight men 1.60 (95% CI 1.09–2.33) and obese men 1.62 (95% CI 1.04–2.53) but this effect was not seen in women. WC was not associated with adenoma recurrence in the total population or in gender specific subgroups. In a larger analysis of 8 trials on 9167 subjects, Martinez and colleagues[24] confirmed a BMI of 30 kg/m^2 or more to be a significant independent risk factor for recurrent adenoma (1.23, 95% CI 1.08–1.41) but not advanced adenoma, compared with individuals with a BMI of less than 25 kg/m^2.

The effect of distribution of adiposity on colorectal neoplasia risk has been assessed in a few studies. The contribution of visceral adiposity to risk as measured by abdomino-pelvic computed tomography (CT) scan, was evaluated in 200 asymptomatic Korean subjects undergoing CT and colonoscopy for routine health evaluation.[25] VAT and WC were significantly higher in those with colorectal neoplasia. The odds ratio of neoplasia was 4.07 (95% CI 1.01–16.43) for those with VAT over 136.61 cm^2 over relative to those with a VAT of less than 67.23 cm^2. WC was not independently associated with colorectal neoplasia. Another Korean case-control study of 165 adenoma cases and 365 polyp-free controls determined that abdominal obesity (as measured at the top of the hip bone by a doctor, and defined by a waist circumference of ≥90 cm for men and ≥85 cm for women) was associated with an increased risk of colorectal adenoma.[26] The association persisted when adjusted for BMI and the strength of the association was similar in men 2.77 (95% CI 1.54–5.00) and women 2.65 (95% CI 1.02–6.90). The prevalence of adenomas and advanced adenomas was 37% and 9% in the abdominally obese group versus 22% and 3% in the normal waist group, respectively.

OTHER EFFECTS OF OBESITY ON THE COLON

Diverticulosis is a common age-related condition. It is estimated that nearly two-thirds of individuals will develop diverticulosis by the age of 85 years although only 15% will experience a serious complication. Two studies have reported on the effects of obesity on the complications of diverticulosis. The first was a small retrospective study of 61 patients that compared the mean BMI in 16 patients who required emergency surgery for perforated diverticulitis, 11 patients admitted with 2 or more episodes of diverticulitis, 16 patients admitted with a single episode of diverticulitis, and 18 individuals with diverticulosis detected on colonoscopy.[27] Although the study has many limitations, not the least of which includes differences in the proportion of men and women and the mean age of individuals in each group, the mean BMI was significantly higher in those with perforation and abscess (32.53 kg/m^2, 95% CI 29.02–36.03) and recurrent diverticulitis (31.91 kg/m^2, 95% CI 29.17–34.64) versus those with a single episode of diverticulosis (25.60 kg/m^2, 95% CI 23.46–27.75) or the diverticulosis controls (25.56 kg/m^2, 95% CI 23.97–27.14).

More recently, data from 47,228 male participants in the Health Professionals Follow-up Study, was analyzed to assess the effect of physical activity on complications of diverticular disease including diverticulitis and bleeding.[28] After 18 years of follow-up the RR for men in the highest quintile of total activity was 0.75 (95% CI 0.58–0.95) for diverticulitis and 0.54 (95% CI 0.38–0.77) for bleeding versus men in the lowest quintile. The decrease in risk was mainly attributable to vigorous physical activity. The risk of complications from diverticular disease associated with physical inactivity was greatest in obese men (BMI $\geq$30 kg/m^2) in the lowest tertile of activity with a RR of 1.62 (95% CI 1.16–2.26) for diverticulitis and 2.81 (95% CI 1.76–4.46) for bleeding for men versus men with a BMI of less than 25 kg/m^2 in the highest tertile of activity.

COLORECTAL CANCER SCREENING

Several studies have assessed the effect of BMI on colorectal cancer screening compliance. One cross-sectional study of 129,000 individuals in the Cancer Prevention Study II Nutritional Cohort found an inverse association between use of screening and BMI.[29] In another study of patients in primary care offices, obese patients had 25% decreased odds of being screened for colorectal cancer compared with nonobese patients (OR 0.75, 95% CI 0.62–0.91).[30] Data from the BRFSS (Behavioral Risk Factor Surveillance System) in 2001 suggested that men in the overweight and obese range were 25% more likely to have undergone a screening sigmoidoscopy within the previous 5 years, whereas women in the obese range were less likely to have undergone a screening sigmoidoscopy compared with women of normal weight.[31] This gender disparity was also confirmed in another study which found colorectal cancer screening rates with fecal occult blood tests or sigmoidoscopy of 45% in nonoverweight men and 45.3% in morbidly obese men.[32] Conversely, rates were 43% in nonoverweight women and 37% in morbidly obese women.

BOWEL PREPARATION

The role of BMI in predicting inadequate bowel preparation was assessed in 1588 patients undergoing colonoscopy.[33] A BMI of 25 kg/m^2 or more was an independent predictor of inadequate preparation and was associated with an inadequate composite score that took into account a subjective bowel preparation score, earlier recommendation for follow-up colonoscopy, and endoscopist confidence in adequate evaluation of the colon and the examination. Each unit increase in BMI increased the likelihood of an inadequate composite score by 2%.

SURGICAL OUTCOMES AFTER LAPAROSCOPIC COLECTOMY FOR COLON CANCER

One hundred and thirty-three consecutive patients undergoing elective laparoscopic sigmoid colectomy for cancer were studied to assess the effect of obesity as measured by VAT or BMI on surgical outcome.[34] VAT was determined by manual tracing of the visceral fat area at the level of the umbilicus on CT scan and considered abnormal if it measured 130 cm^2 or more. A BMI of 25 kg/m^2 or more was considered obese. Patients characterized as obese by VAT, but not by BMI, had a higher incidence of wound infection (21% vs 5%), overall complication rates (32% vs 12%), and a longer postoperative hospital stay (10.5 vs 9 days) than nonobese patients.

SUMMARY

Obesity is a risk factor for colorectal cancer and adenomatous polyps. The adequate detection of neoplasia may be hampered by a suboptimal bowel preparation in obese patients who undergo colonoscopy. Some studies have shown variable risk estimates for neoplasia by gender, cancer location, and fat distribution; visceral adipose tissue has a particularly increased association. The complex metabolic activity of adipose tissue results in the production of proinflammatory cytokines and neurohumoral and immune-mediated mechanisms leading to systemic effects including insulin resistance. These adverse effects of obesity on the colon promote carcinogenesis, seem to impair wound healing and repair, and may be ameliorated by enhanced physical activity, weight loss, or increased muscular strength.

REFERENCES

1. Calle EE, Thun M, Petrelli JM, et al. Body-mass index and mortality in a prospective cohort of U.S. Adults. N Engl J Med 1995;341:1097–105.
2. Pischon T, Boeing H, Hoffman K, et al. General and abdominal adiposity and risk of death in Europe. N Engl J Med 2008;359:2105–20.
3. Executive summary of the clinical guidelines on the identification, evaluation, and treatment of overweight and obesity in adults. Arch Intern Med 1998;158(17): 1855–67.
4. American Cancer Society. Cancer facts and figures 2003. New York: American Cancer Society; 2003.
5. Gunter MJ, Leitzmann MF. Obesity and colorectal cancer: epidemiology, mechanisms and candidate genes. J Nutr Biochem 2006;17:145–6.
6. Jones ME, McInnes KJ, Boon WC, et al. Estrogen and adiposity. Utilizing models of aromatase deficiency to explore the relationship. J Steroid Biochem Mol Biol 2007;106:3–7.
7. Fenton JI, Lavigne JA, Perkins SN, et al. Microarray analysis reveals that leptin induces autocrine/paracrine cascades to promote survival and proliferation of colon epithelial cells in an Apc genotype-dependant fashion. Mol Carcinog 2008;47:9–21.
8. Abolhassani M, Aloulou N, Chaumetter MT, et al. Leptin-receptor-related immune response in colorectal tumors: the role of colonocytes and interleukin-8. Cancer Res 2008;68:9423–32.
9. Aloulou N, Bastuji-Garin S, Le Gouvello S, et al. Involvement of the leptin receptor in the immune response in intestinal cancer. Cancer Res 2008;68:9413–22.
10. dos Santos LC, de Padua Cintra I, Fisberg M, et al. Calcium intake and its relationship with adiposity and insulin resistance in post-pubertal adolescents. J Hum Nutr Diet 2008;21:109–16.
11. Harris SS, Dawson-Hughes B. Reduced sun exposure does not explain the inverse association of 25-hydroxyvitamin D with percent body fat in older adults. J Clin Endocrinol Metab 2007;92:3155–7.
12. Adams KF, Leitzmann MF, Ablanes D, et al. Body mass and colorectal cancer risk in the NIH-AARP cohort. Am J Epidemiol 2007;166:36–45.
13. Ford ES. Body mass index and colon cancer in a national sample of adult US men and women. Am J Epidemiol 1999;150:390–6.
14. Moore LL, Bradlee ML, Singer MR, et al. BMI and waist circumference as predictors of lifetime colon cancer risk in Framingham study adults. Int J Obes 2004;28:559–67.

15. Pischon T, Lahmann PH, Boeing H, et al. Body size and risk of colon and rectal cancer in the European prospective investigation into cancer and nutrition (EPIC). J Natl Cancer Inst 2006;98:920–31.

16. Moghaddam AA, Woodward M, Huxley R. Obesity and risk of colorectal cancer: a meta-analysis of 31 studies with 70,000 events. Cancer Epidemiol Biomarkers Prev 2007;16:2533–47.

17. Larsson SC, Wolk A. Obesity and colon and rectal cancer risk: a meta-analysis of prospective studies. Am J Clin Nutr 2007;86:556–65.

18. Ruiz JR, Sui X, Lobelo F, et al. Muscular strength and adiposity as predictors of adulthood cancer mortality n men. Cancer Epidemiol Biomarkers Prev 2009;18: 1468–76.

19. Wei EK, Ma J, Pollak MN, et al. C-peptide, insulin like growth factor binding protein-1, glycosolated hemoglobin, and the risk of distal colorectal adenoma in women. Cancer Epidemiol Biomarkers Prev 2006;15:750–5.

20. Yamaji Y, Okamoto M, Yoshida H, et al. The effect of body weight reduction on the incidence of colorectal adenoma. Am J Gastroenterol 2008;103:2061–7.

21. Sedjo RL, Byers T, Levin TR, et al. Change in body size and the risk of colorectal adenomas. Cancer Epidemiol Biomarkers Prev 2007;16(3):526–31.

22. Wise LA, Rosenberg L, Palmer JR, et al. Anthropometric risk factors for colorectal polyps in African American women. Obesity (Silver Spring) 2008;16:859–68.

23. Jacobs ET, Martinez ME, Alberts DS, et al. Association between body size and colorectal adenoma recurrence. Clin Gastroenterol Hepatol 2007;5:982–90.

24. Martinez ME, Baron JA, Lieberman DA, et al. A pooled analysis of advanced colorectal neoplasia diagnoses after colonoscopic polypectomy. Gastroenterology 2009;136:832–41.

25. Oh TH, Byeon JS, Myung SJ, et al. Visceral obesity as a risk factor for colorectal neoplasm. J Gastroenterol Hepatol 2008;23:411–7.

26. Kim Y, Kim Y, Lee S. An association between colonic adenoma and abdominal obesity: a cross sectional study. BMC Gastroenterol 2009;9:410/1186/1471-230X-9-4.

27. Dobbins C, DeFontgalland D, Duthie G, et al. The relationship of obesity to the complications of diverticular disease. Colorectal Dis 2005;8:37–40.

28. Strate LL, Liu YL, Aldoori W, et al. Physical activity decreases diverticular complications. Am J Gastroenterol 2009;104:1221–30.

29. Chao A, Connell CJ, Cokkinides V, et al. Underuse of screening sigmoidoscopy and colonoscopy n a large cohort of US adults. Am J Public Health 2004;94: 1775–81.

30. Ferrante JM, Ohman-Strickland P, Hudson SV, et al. Colorectal cancer screening among obese versus non-obese patients in primary care practices. Cancer Detect Prev 2006;30:459–65.

31. Heo M, Allison DB, Fontaine KB. Overweight, obesity, and colorectal cancer screening: disparity between men and women. BMC Public Health 2004;4:53–8.

32. Rosen AB, Schneider EC. Colorectal cancer screening disparities related to obesity and gender. J Gen Intern Med 2004;19:332–8.

33. Borg BB, Gupta NK, Zuckerman GR, et al. Impact of obesity on bowel preparation for colonoscopy. Clin Gastroenterol Hepatol 2009;7:670–5.

34. Tsujinaka S, Konishi F, Kawamura YJ, et al. Viscreal obesity predicts surgical outcomes after laparoscopic colectomy for sigmoid colon cancer. Dis Colon Rectum 2008;51:1757–67.

Hepatic Complications of Obesity

Anna Mae Diehl, MD

KEYWORDS

- Nonalcoholic fatty liver disease • Steatohepatitis
- Cirrhosis • Hepatocellular carcinoma

Obesity is associated with a spectrum of chronic liver disease. Hepatic steatosis (fatty liver) is an appropriate physiologic response to excessive calories. Hence, fatty liver is common because obesity is common. Some individuals with hepatic steatosis develop steatohepatitis, a more serious form of liver damage that may lead to progressive fibrosis, and ultimately to cirrhosis. As with cirrhosis caused by habitual alcohol abuse or chronic viral hepatitis, cirrhosis related to obesity can be complicated by primary liver cancer, both hepatocellular carcinoma and intrahepatic cholangiocarcinoma. Primary liver cancers have also been demonstrated in patients with steatohepatitis who have not yet become cirrhotic, although this seems to occur relatively infrequently. Because obesity increases the risk for advanced forms of liver disease (ie, cirrhosis and liver cancer), the obesity epidemic is emerging as a major factor underlying the burden of liver disease in the United States and many other countries. This article reviews mechanisms that mediate the pathogenesis of obesity-related liver disease, summarizes clinical evidence that demonstrates that obesity-related liver disease can be life-threatening, and discusses whether or not treatments for obesity or related comorbidities impact liver disease outcomes.

HISTOPATHOLOGY AND PATHOGENESIS OF OBESITY-RELATED LIVER DISEASE

Obesity is associated with a spectrum of fatty liver diseases, the most common of which is hepatic steatosis (fatty liver).[1] Population-based studies that relied on sensitive abdominal imaging techniques to detect hepatic triglyceride demonstrate that about a third of the United States adult population has hepatic steatosis.[2] In those studies, fatty liver was strongly associated with obesity. Other risk factors include insulin resistance and dyslipidemia, conditions that are also extremely prevalent in the general population. Although fatty liver disease may also occur in nonobese individuals, including those with lipoatrophy[3] or who consume excessive alcohol,[4] overweight-obesity remains one of the greatest risk factors for fatty liver disease.

Department of Medicine, Division of Gastroenterology, Duke University, Snyderman Building, Suite 1073, Durham, NC 27710, USA
E-mail address: diehl004@mc.duke.edu

Gastroenterol Clin N Am 39 (2010) 57–68
doi:10.1016/j.gtc.2009.12.001
0889-8553/10/$ – see front matter © 2010 Elsevier Inc. All rights reserved.

gastro.theclinics.com

Fatty liver is associated with obesity because the liver responds to caloric excess by synthesizing triglyceride. Normally, these triglycerides are then exported from the liver in lipoproteins and stored in peripheral adipose depots. Triglycerides are retained in the liver when their assimilation into peripheral adipose tissues is impaired or when lipoprotein export mechanisms become inefficient. Systemic insulin resistance is a common cause of the former, whereas various conditions that interfere with efficient packaging and secretion of lipoproteins from hepatocytes (eg, abetalipoproteinemia, choline deficiency) cause the latter.[5]

Based on analysis of case series at referral centers, it is estimated that about a quarter of the individuals with fatty livers have steatohepatitis.[6] Steatohepatitis is a more serious form of liver damage than simple steatosis because hepatocyte injury or death is significantly more prominent in steatohepatitis than in simple steatosis, and this hepatic injury is often accompanied by inflammatory cell accumulation and some degree of fibrosis.[7] Obesity-related steatohepatitis resembles alcohol-induced steatohepatitis histologically, and obesity seems to increase the risk of developing alcohol-induced fatty liver.[8] Hence, a clinical diagnosis of nonalcoholic steatohepatitis (NASH) can only be made when it is certain that there has been less than or equal to only social levels of alcohol consumption (ie, ≤2 drinks per day).[9]

Analysis of groups of nonalcoholic patients who have undergone sequential liver biopsies suggests that as many as a third of NASH patients may progress to cirrhosis within a decade of follow-up,[6] whereas progressive fibrosis rarely occurs in patients who merely have steatosis on index liver biopsy.[10] In NASH, as in most other causes of chronic hepatitis, the risk of progressing to cirrhosis is greatest in patients who demonstrate fibrosis on their initial liver biopsy.[11] Like patients with other types of chronic fibrosing liver diseases, patients with NASH develop bridging fibrosis as cirrhosis evolves.[12] NASH is also characterized by a unique pattern of collagen deposition around hepatocytes and along sinusoids, however, even relatively early stages of liver injury.[13] This pericellular-perisinusoidal fibrosis is presumably part of a wound-healing response to ongoing liver injury.[14] It is typically most prominent in the areas of the liver lobule that are near terminal hepatic venules (zone 3), where hepatocyte injury begins in NASH, and has been dubbed "chicken wire fibrosis."[15] Although a subset of individuals with NASH develop progressive liver fibrosis and ultimately become cirrhotic over time, others remain stable and still others improve.[16] At present, the factors that determine the outcomes of NASH are not well understood.

Emerging evidence also suggests that primary liver cancers, both hepatocellular carcinoma and intrahepatic cholangiocarcinoma, can occur during NASH.[17] Fortunately, this seems to be a relatively rare occurrence until cirrhosis is well-established.[18] Cirrhosis remains the more common underlying liver disorder in obese patients with primary hepatic neoplasms. It has been estimated that the risk of developing primary liver cancer is about 1% per year once cirrhosis has developed in NASH.

CLINICAL FEATURES AND LABORATORY ABNORMALITIES OF OBESITY-RELATED LIVER DISEASES

Liver disease often goes undetected for decades in obese individuals because serum aminotransferase values may be normal or only mildly elevated on an intermittent basis. As in other liver diseases, hyperbilirubinemia (jaundice), hypoalbuminemia, and coagulopathy develop only when liver damage is very advanced. In addition, abdominal adiposity may compromise early diagnosis of hepatomegaly or more subtle abnormalities related to portal hypertension (ie, splenomegaly, ascites).[19] Individuals with obesity-related liver disease typically exhibit an android pattern of adiposity (ie, relative overexpansion of abdominal adipose depots) and clinical features of insulin resistance (eg, acanthosis nigricans, polycystic ovary syndrome).[20] They also often have laboratory abnormalities that are characteristic of the metabolic syndrome, including hypercholesterolemia; low levels of high-density lipoproteins; hypertriglceridemia; hyperuricemia; hyperinsulinemia; insulin resistance on glucose tolerance testing; and even fasting hyperglycemia (ie, diabetes).[21] Serum levels of autoantibodies, such as antinuclear antibody or anti–smooth muscle antibody, may be increased, but elevated levels of total serum proteins rarely occur and hyperglobulinemia is not typical unless cirrhosis with portal-systemic shunting has already developed.[22] Hyperferritinemia in the absence of other evidence of iron overload (ie, transferrin saturation or increased serum iron concentration) has been reported to occur in some patients with obesity-related fatty liver disease.[23,24] Markers for chronic viral hepatitis, Wilson disease, and α_1-antitrypsin deficiency, however, are typically negative.[9] Abdominal imaging studies generally demonstrate hepatic steatosis, although different approaches differ in their sensitivity for detecting hepatic fat.[25] Proton nuclear magnetic resonance spectroscopy is the most sensitive technique, but this is not widely applied outside of research settings. Comparison of liver-spleen density on either standard MRI or CT is generally useful. Routine ultrasonography (the least sensitive test) is capable of detecting hepatic fat when accumulation is present in more than a third of the liver cells. Because there is no one serum marker that is diagnostic of fatty liver disease and fatty liver is an extremely prevalent condition, testing must be done to exclude other causes of chronic aminotransferase elevations before concluding that steatosis-NASH is the explanation for abnormal liver enzymes when fatty liver has been demonstrated by some type of abdominal imaging study.[9]

It is also important to emphasize that the magnitude of aminotransferase elevation is not reliable for distinguishing NASH from steatosis. Serum liver enzymes can be normal in individuals with NASH or NASH-related cirrhosis and may be increased in individuals with simple steatosis.[26] Recently, it has been suggested that serum levels of cytokeratin 8/18 cleavage products (which are produced during cellular apoptosis) are generally greater in NASH than in simple steatosis and may be helpful in differentiating individuals with NASH (who have a more ominous prognosis) from those with steatosis (who are likely to follow a benign clinical course).[27] Combinations of clinical tests (eg, the AST/ALT ratio plus platelet count) or commercially available fibrosis markers are also somewhat helpful in identifying patients who are developing liver fibrosis.[28,29] At present, however, liver biopsy remains the gold standard test for confirming the clinical suspicion of NASH, for grading the severity of resultant liver injury and inflammation, and for establishing the stage of fibrosis.[30,31] As in other types of chronic liver disease, in NASH the accuracy of liver biopsy for staging the extent of liver fibrosis depends on the size of the biopsy core, and sampling artifacts may be problematic in biopsy specimens that are less than 2 cm in length.[32,33]

COMORBID CONDITIONS COMMONLY ASSOCIATED WITH OBESITY-RELATED LIVER DISEASE

Obesity-related liver disease is strongly associated with certain other medical conditions. These include insulin resistance and type 2 diabetes; dyslipidemias hypercholesterolemia, low high-density lipoprotein, hypertriglyceridemia, and hypertension (ie, the metabolic syndrome); polycystic ovary syndrome; cardiovascular disease; cancers; sleep apnea; and hypothyroidism. It has been difficult to determine which, if any, of these conditions contribute to the pathogenesis of nonalcoholic fatty live and NASH and which comorbidities are actually consequences of the liver pathology. Preclinical and clinical research suggests that insulin resistance is involved in the pathogenesis of nonalcoholic fatty liver and NASH.[34,35] It has also been postulated that sleep apnea causes hypoxia and stress-related hormonal responses that may contribute to the severity of fatty liver injury.[36] Chronic liver injury may provoke activation of tissue deiodinases that inactivate thyroid hormones, however, thereby promoting hypothyroidism.[37] Recently, hypothyroidism was identified as an independent risk factor for hepatocellular carcinoma in women.[38] Chronic liver injury probably also contributes to systemic inflammation that is now believed to fuel progressive cardiovascular disease, exacerbate insulin resistance, and increase the risk for various types of malignancy.[39] Sex hormones also seem to influence the prevalence and severity of fatty liver disease.[40] Hepatic steatosis is generally more common in men than women, but nonalcoholic fatty liver disease (NAFLD)-related cirrhosis seems to occur more often in women. Among women with fatty liver disease, disease severity seems to worsen after menopause.[41] Certain ethnic groups are also more vulnerable to fatty liver damage than others. For example, studies suggest that risk is greatest in Asians and Native Americans (including Hispanics and Eskimos), intermediate in whites, and lowest in African Americans.[2]

PROGNOSIS OF OBESITY-RELATED LIVER DISEASE

Population-based studies demonstrate that fatty liver disease increases both overall and liver-related mortality.[42] As in the general population, cardiovascular disease is the leading cause of death in patients with NAFLD. Moreover, the severity of NAFLD-related liver injury seems to influence the risk for mortality from cardiovascular disease: death from cardiovascular disease is lower in individuals who do not have fatty livers than in those who do, and higher in patients with NASH than in those with simple steatosis.[30] Cancer is the second leading cause of death in NAFLD patients, as it is in the general adult population.[4,42] Liver disease is the third leading cause of mortality in NAFLD patients, however, whereas it ranks as the eighteenth leading cause of death in adults without fatty livers.[42]

Because NAFLD is more than an order of magnitude more prevalent in the United States than chronic viral hepatitis, NAFLD is the most common cause of cirrhosis in American adults,[43] despite the fact that progression to cirrhosis probably occurs in fewer than 5% of the NAFLD population.[4,44] Head-to-head comparison of outcomes in patients with cirrhosis related to either chronic hepatitis C or NAFLD has revealed that both types of liver disease have similarly ominous outcomes, including significant morbidity and mortality related to portal hypertension, liver failure, or primary liver cancer.[45] Indeed, because the diagnosis of cirrhosis tends to be delayed in NAFLD compared with chronic hepatitis C, NAFLD patients are more likely to present to physicians with complications of advanced liver disease (eg, ascites, variceal hemorrhage, hepatocellular carcinoma) than patients with hepatitis C virus–related cirrhosis, who are typically diagnosed before overt symptoms and signs of liver disease emerge.[46] Also, comorbidities and older age often preclude consideration of liver transplantation as a treatment option for patients with NAFLD-cirrhosis, rendering many of these patients dependent on medical management of hepatic decompensation.[47]

EFFECTS OF WEIGHT LOSS AND TREATING COMORBIDITIES ON LIVER DISEASE OUTCOMES

The ultimate objective of therapy for obesity-related fatty liver disease is to prevent progression to cirrhosis. In addition, management must include efforts to prevent adverse outcomes from associated cardiovascular disease and cancer, which are the top two causes of death in this patient population. Because cardiovascular disease, cancer, and cirrhosis are all ultimately complications of obesity, weight reduction is a primary therapeutic target.[48] Success requires consistent reductions in energy intake relative to energy expenditure. This can be accomplished either by caloric restriction (diet); increased exercise; or combinations of these two approaches. At present, there is not consistent evidence that restricting one particular type of macronutrient (ie, dietary fats or carbohydrate) provides benefit beyond what is realized when total calorie ingestion is reduced.[49] Similarly, because the major benefits of exercise seem to be related to its effects on net energy expenditure with resultant reduction in overall adiposity, the level of physical activity must be sufficiently vigorous and sustained to provoke catabolism. This generally necessitates at least 30 minutes of moderately aerobic exercise five times per week. Obese patients with NAFLD often find it difficult to achieve these goals because they tend to be very physically deconditioned.[50] Hence, diet generally becomes the mainstay of therapy, although an exercise program that includes a combination of aerobic and resistance work should be encouraged.

Weight reduction medications, such as drugs that enhance fat malabsorption, have not been proved to provide benefits beyond that achieved alone by caloric restriction.[51] Recently, clinical trials with cannabinoid receptor 1 (CB1) antagonists were initiated because in addition to their anorexogenic actions, these drugs seemed to improve insulin sensitivity and prevent liver fibrosis in preclinical studies. The trials in humans were halted, however, because of major neuropsychiatric adverse events that were associated with chronic use of CB1 antagonists.

Bariatric surgery is another approach that is often considered to improve obesity. It is extremely effective in accomplishing long-term reductions in body mass index and improves many of the comorbidities that accompany obesity, including hypertension, dyslipidemia, sleep apnea, and insulin resistance.[52] Indeed, the latter improves dramatically within days of surgery, long before significant weight loss is observed, suggesting that some of the benefits of bariatric surgery may be mediated by changes in gut-derived neuropeptides.[53] Noncirrhotic patients with NAFLD generally tolerate bariatric surgery without added morbidity or mortality and seem to respond with reductions in hepatic steatosis and necroinflammation.[54] Long-term effects on liver fibrosis remain uncertain because follow-up liver biopsies have not been done routinely.[55,56] Cirrhosis remains a general contraindication to bariatric surgery, as it is to most types of elective intra-abdominal surgical procedures, because of the increased risk for perioperative hepatic decompensation and liver-related mortality. At present, comparative data on the relative merits of different types of bariatric surgical procedures on liver histology are scant, but it seems likely that the greatest reductions in hepatic steatosis will result from those procedures that produce the greatest and most sustained reductions in body mass index.[57]

Obese patients with NAFLD typically have comorbid illnesses. Evidence proves that treating these conditions is generally not harmful to the liver. Indeed, in some circumstances, it may actually help to improve fatty liver disease.[58] Postmarketing surveillance of statin treatment for hypercholesterolemia, for example, demonstrates that (contrary to expectations) statin therapy is associated with improvements in liver enzyme elevations in NAFLD patients.[59] Prospective, controlled trials to evaluate the efficacy of statins as a therapy for NASH have not been reported. Small case series suggest, however, that statins may improve steatosis and hepatic inflammation.[60] Effects on liver fibrosis have not yet been established.[61] Fibrate therapy for hypertriglycerdemia also seems to be harmless for the liver, but there is no evidence that these agents actually improve NASH.[62] Data from a growing number of clinical trials suggest, however, that several different insulin-sensitizing agents that are used to treat diabetes may also improve NASH (see later). Certain cardiovascular therapeutics, such as angiotensin receptor blockers, have also been evaluated as treatments for NASH, and seem to reduce both hepatic necroinflammatory activity and liver fibrosis in small, nonrandomized studies.[63] Replacing thyroid hormones to normalize serum levels of free T4 is not known to harm (or independently benefit) the underlying fatty liver disease. Treatment of sleep apnea with continuous positive airway pressure has been shown to improve nocturnal hypoxemia and reduce related stress responses that may contribute to weight gain, hypertension, and cardiac dysfunction, but it remains to be proved that these apparent benefits of continuous positive airway pressure prevent or improve NASH.

TARGETED PHARMACOLOGIC TREATMENTS FOR OBESITY-RELATED LIVER DISEASE

As in most types of chronic liver disease, in obesity-related liver disease, liver-related morbidity and mortality is largely restricted to individuals who develop cirrhosis. The goal of treatment is to prevent cirrhosis. This might be accomplished by preventing individuals with "simple" hepatic steatosis from developing NASH, because cirrhosis rarely occurs without antecedent NASH. Given the high prevalence of fatty liver in the general population and evidence that only a relatively small subset (approximately 25%) of these individuals develop NASH, however, the risk/benefit ratio of such treatment needs to be very high and the cost of therapy very low. In addition, the relatively low incidence of NASH (and subsequent cirrhosis) suggests that large numbers of subjects need to be followed prospectively for many years to establish the true benefits of putative NASH-preventing therapies.

Given these constraints, most investigators have deployed a second strategy to prevent NAFLD-related cirrhosis (ie, improving NASH in patients who have already developed this condition). To establish efficacy, such studies require initial proof of NASH. Liver histology is a criterion for enrollment. End-of-treatment liver histology is also essential because changes in the severity of NASH are not reliably assessed by existing serologic markers or abdominal imaging. Placebo-treated controls must also be included to ensure that the rate of NASH regression in the study group exceeds that which is known to occur "spontaneously."[16] Ideally, subjects are followed long enough to determine if improvements in histologic parameters of NASH (hepatic steatosis, liver cell injury or death, hepatic inflammation) reduce or prevent liver fibrosis. Because only about 20% of NASH patients develop bridging fibrosis or cirrhosis within a decade of initial liver biopsy,[9] relatively large sample size and lengthy duration of follow-up are required to prove that improvements in NASH actually translate into cirrhosis prevention. It is also important to demonstrate that benefits for the liver are achieved without inadvertently exacerbating other potentially life-threatening comorbidities, such as cardiovascular disease and cancer.

Very few, if any, of the published clinical trials for NAFLD therapies have fulfilled all of these desirable metrics. Most were small, nonrandomized studies with relatively short durations of follow-up. Some did not require liver histology for enrollment, whereas others relied on surrogate markers of liver injury, rather than histology, to assess treatment effects. These limitations confound efforts to judge the putative merits of antioxidants (eg, vitamin E, betaine),[64–69] angiotensin receptor antagonists (losartan),[63,70] and metformin[71–73] in NASH. A multicenter, prospective, placebo-controlled trial was unable to demonstrate that treatment with ursodeoxycholic acid was superior to placebo in improving NASH,[74] despite earlier suggestions that this agent might be beneficial. More recent, small studies of other bile salt–like agents[75] or combination therapy with ursodeoxycholic acid and vitamin E[76] have suggested that bile salts might have efficacy. Hence, the ultimate role of bile salt–like agents as NASH therapies remains to be determined. Also uncertain is the role of prebiotics or probiotics as potential treatments for NASH.[77,78] Such agents are intriguing because they are generally safe and relatively inexpensive and might correct obesity-related alterations in the intestinal microbiome that may contribute to obesity, insulin resistance, and hepatic inflammation.[79] Caspase inhibitors are also being considered as possible treatments for NASH[80] to reduce hepatocyte apoptosis (which is increased in NASH)[81] back toward more normal levels. Inhibiting programmed cell death in NASH patients, who are at generally increased risk for cancer, however, prompts at least theoretical concern. Finally, preclinical studies suggest that drugs that modulate cannabinoid receptor activity (either CB1 antagonists or CB2 agonists)[82] or that increase the actions of sirtuins (eg, resveratrol)[83] might also be useful in NASH. At this point, however, clinical data on their efficacy is extremely limited.

In contrast to all of these other agents, thiazolidinediones (TZDs) have been fairly extensively examined as treatments for NASH. TZDs have insulin-sensitizing and anti-inflammatory actions and interest in them as potential treatments for NASH has been driven by evidence that insulin resistance and chronic inflammation play important roles in NASH pathogenesis.[84] To date, results have been reported from several human studies, and statistically beneficial effects on steatosis and liver necroinflammation were demonstrated after treatment with troglitazone, rosiglitazone, or pioglitazone.[85–88] Benefits were observed only during drug therapy, however, and quickly subsided when treatment was withdrawn. In addition, liver histology did not improve in all of the TZD-treated subjects in any trial, despite generalized treatment-related improvements in insulin sensitivity. Therapy also tended to be associated with weight gain. Most importantly, improvement in liver fibrosis was not observed consistently, even in subjects who were continued on TZD therapy and re-evaluated 3 years later.[89] Hence, the ultimate efficacy of TZDs in preventing cirrhosis remains uncertain. This tempers enthusiasm for recommending long-term therapy with these agents simply to prevent progressive liver disease. Caution is particularly justified given recent evidence that one of the TZDs (rosiglitazone) might increase cardiovascular mortality,[90] because this is the leading cause of death in NASH patients.

SUMMARY

Obesity often leads to hepatic steatosis. Some obese patients with hepatic steatosis develop a more serious liver damage, dubbed "nonalcoholic steatohepatitis." Although NASH can regress, some patients with NASH eventually develop cirrhosis or primary liver cancer. Liver-related morbidity and mortality occur mainly in cirrhotic patients. Liver disease is the third leading cause of death in such individuals, who also exhibit increased risk of death from cardiovascular disease and cancer. Hence, the main goal of treatment for obesity-related liver disease is to prevent cirrhosis without exacerbating cardiovascular disease or promoting carcinogenesis. Growing knowledge about the mechanisms involved in the pathogenesis of NASH suggests several potential therapies for this disease. Only one class of drug (ie, TZDs) has been widely investigated as a treatment for NASH. TZD therapy improves certain histologic features of NASH in some, but not all, patients. More importantly, there is not yet compelling evidence that sustained TZD therapy prevents (or improves) liver fibrosis. More research is needed to identify treatments that prevent patients with NASH from developing cirrhosis and resultant liver-related morbidity and mortality. There is strong evidence that weight reduction and treating obesity-related comorbidities (eg, dyslipidemia, hypertension, diabetes, hypothyroidism, sleep apnea) is safe and, perhaps, beneficial for the underlying liver condition.

REFERENCES

1. Angulo P. Obesity and nonalcoholic fatty liver disease. Nutr Rev 2007;65(6 Pt 2): S57–63.
2. Browning JD, Szczepaniak LS, Dobbins R, et al. Prevalence of hepatic steatosis in an urban population in the United States: impact of ethnicity. Hepatology 2004; 40(6):1387–95.
3. Bingham A, Mamyrova G, Rother KI, et al. Predictors of acquired lipodystrophy in juvenile-onset dermatomyositis and a gradient of severity. Medicine (Baltimore) 2008;87(2):70–86.
4. Dam-Larsen S, Becker U, Franzmann MB, et al. Final results of a long-term, clinical follow-up in fatty liver patients. Scand J Gastroenterol 2009;44(10): 1236–43.
5. Choi SS, Diehl AM. Hepatic triglyceride synthesis and nonalcoholic fatty liver disease. Curr Opin Lipidol 2008;19(3):295–300.
6. Matteoni CA, Younossi ZM, Gramlich T, et al. Nonalcoholic fatty liver disease: a spectrum of clinical and pathological severity. Gastroenterology 1999;116(6): 1413–9.
7. Yeh MM, Brunt EM. Pathology of nonalcoholic fatty liver disease. Am J Clin Pathol 2007;128(5):837–47.
8. Bellentani S, Saccoccio G, Masutti F, et al. Prevalence of and risk factors for hepatic steatosis in Northern Italy. Ann Intern Med 2000;132(2):112–7.
9. McCullough AJ. The clinical features, diagnosis and natural history of nonalcoholic fatty liver disease. Clin Liver Dis 2004;8(3):521–33, viii.
10. Teli MR, James OF, Burt AD, et al. The natural history of nonalcoholic fatty liver: a follow-up study. Hepatology 1995;22(6):1714–9.
11. Feldstein AE, Papouchado BG, Angulo P, et al. Hepatic stellate cells and fibrosis progression in patients with nonalcoholic fatty liver disease. Clin Gastroenterol Hepatol 2005;3(4):384–9.
12. Richardson MM, Jonsson JR, Powell EE, et al. Progressive fibrosis in nonalcoholic steatohepatitis: association with altered regeneration and a ductular reaction. Gastroenterology 2007;133(1):80–90.
13. Gramlich T, Kleiner DE, McCullough AJ, et al. Pathologic features associated with fibrosis in nonalcoholic fatty liver disease. Hum Pathol 2004;35(2):196–9.
14. Jou J, Choi SS, Diehl AM. Mechanisms of disease progression in nonalcoholic fatty liver disease. Semin Liver Dis 2008;28(4):370–9.
15. Lefkowitch JH. Morphology of alcoholic liver disease. Clin Liver Dis 2005;9(1): 37–53.
16. Adams LA, Sanderson S, Lindor KD, et al. The histological course of nonalcoholic fatty liver disease: a longitudinal study of 103 patients with sequential liver biopsies. J Hepatol 2005;42(1):132–8.
17. Hashizume H, Sato K, Takagi H, et al. Primary liver cancers with nonalcoholic steatohepatitis. Eur J Gastroenterol Hepatol 2007;19(10):827–34.
18. Siegel AB, Zhu AX. Metabolic syndrome and hepatocellular carcinoma: two growing epidemics with a potential link. Cancer 2009;115(24):5651–61.
19. Ratziu V, Giral P, Charlotte F, et al. Liver fibrosis in overweight patients. Gastroenterology 2000;118(6):1117–23.

20. Vega GL, Chandalia M, Szczepaniak LS, et al. Metabolic correlates of nonalcoholic fatty liver in women and men. Hepatology 2007;46(3):716–22.
21. Bellentani S, Marino M. Epidemiology and natural history of non-alcoholic fatty liver disease (NAFLD). Ann Hepatol 2009;8(Suppl 1):S4–8.
22. Adams LA, Lindor KD, Angulo P. The prevalence of autoantibodies and autoimmune hepatitis in patients with nonalcoholic fatty liver disease. Am J Gastroenterol 2004;99(7):1316–20.
23. Fargion S, Mattioli M, Fracanzani AL, et al. Hyperferritinemia, iron overload, and multiple metabolic alterations identify patients at risk for nonalcoholic steatohepatitis. Am J Gastroenterol 2001;96(8):2448–55.
24. Yoneda M, Nozaki Y, Endo H, et al. Serum ferritin is a clinical biomarker in Japanese patients with nonalcoholic steatohepatitis (NASH) independent of HFE gene mutation. Dig Dis Sci 2009. [Epub ahead of print].
25. Ma X, Holalkere NS, Kambadakone RA, et al. Imaging-based quantification of hepatic fat: methods and clinical applications. Radiographics 2009;29(5):1253–77.
26. Mofrad P, Contos MJ, Haque M, et al. Clinical and histologic spectrum of nonalcoholic fatty liver disease associated with normal ALT values. Hepatology 2003;37(6):1286–92.
27. Yilmaz Y. Systematic review: caspase-cleaved fragments of cytokeratin 18-the promises and challenges of a biomarker for chronic liver disease. Aliment Pharmacol Ther 2009;30(11–12):1103–9.
28. Ratziu V, Giral P, Munteanu M, et al. Screening for liver disease using non-invasive biomarkers (FibroTest, SteatoTest and NashTest) in patients with hyperlipidaemia. Aliment Pharmacol Ther 2007;25(2):207–18.
29. Wieckowska A, McCullough AJ, Feldstein AE. Noninvasive diagnosis and monitoring of nonalcoholic steatohepatitis: present and future. Hepatology 2007;46(2):582–9.
30. Wieckowska A, Feldstein AE. Diagnosis of nonalcoholic fatty liver disease: invasive versus noninvasive. Semin Liver Dis 2008;28(4):386–95.
31. Angulo P. Noninvasive assessment of fibrosis and steatosis in NASH and ASH. Gastroenterol Clin Biol 2009;33(10–11):940–8.
32. Arun J, Jhala N, Lazenby AJ, et al. Influence of liver biopsy heterogeneity and diagnosis of nonalcoholic steatohepatitis in subjects undergoing gastric bypass. Obes Surg 2007;17(2):155–61.
33. Ratziu V, Charlotte F, Heurtier A, et al. Sampling variability of liver biopsy in nonalcoholic fatty liver disease. Gastroenterology 2005;128(7):1898–906.
34. Marchesini G, Brizi M, Bianchi G, et al. Nonalcoholic fatty liver disease: a feature of the metabolic syndrome. Diabetes 2001;50(8):1844–50.
35. Gholam PM, Flancbaum L, Machan JT, et al. Nonalcoholic fatty liver disease in severely obese subjects. Am J Gastroenterol 2007;102(2):399–408.
36. Mishra P, Nugent C, Afendy A, et al. Apnoeic-hypopnoeic episodes during obstructive sleep apnoea are associated with histological nonalcoholic steatohepatitis. Liver Int 2008;28(8):1080–6.
37. Liangpunsakul S, Chalasani N. Is hypothyroidism a risk factor for non-alcoholic steatohepatitis? J Clin Gastroenterol 2003;37(4):340–3.
38. Hassan MM, Kaseb A, Li D, et al. Association between hypothyroidism and hepatocellular carcinoma: a case-control study in the United States. Hepatology 2009;49(5):1563–70.
39. Kamada Y, Takehara T, Hayashi N. Adipocytokines and liver disease. J Gastroenterol 2008;43(11):811–22.

40. Denzer C, Thiere D, Muche R, et al. Gender-specific prevalences of fatty liver in obese children and adolescents: roles of body fat distribution, sex steroids, and insulin resistance. J Clin Endocrinol Metab 2009;94(10):3872–81.

41. Suzuki A, Abdelmalek MF. Nonalcoholic fatty liver disease in women. Womens Health (Lond Engl) 2009;5(2):191–203.

42. Adams LA, Lymp JF, St Sauver J, et al. The natural history of nonalcoholic fatty liver disease: a population-based cohort study. Gastroenterology 2005;129(1):113–21.

43. Adams LA, Lindor KD. Nonalcoholic fatty liver disease. Ann Epidemiol 2007; 17(11):863–9.

44. Erickson SK. Nonalcoholic fatty liver disease. J Lipid Res 2009;50(Suppl): S412–6.

45. Sanyal AJ, Banas C, Sargeant C, et al. Similarities and differences in outcomes of cirrhosis due to nonalcoholic steatohepatitis and hepatitis C. Hepatology 2006; 43(4):682–9.

46. Ratziu V, Bonyhay L, Di Martino V, et al. Survival, liver failure, and hepatocellular carcinoma in obesity-related cryptogenic cirrhosis. Hepatology 2002;35(6): 1485–93.

47. Burke A, Lucey MR. Non-alcoholic fatty liver disease, non-alcoholic steatohepatitis and orthotopic liver transplantation. Am J Transplant 2004;4(5):686–93.

48. Cortez-Pinto H, Machado M. Impact of body weight, diet and lifestyle on nonalcoholic fatty liver disease. Expert Rev Gastroenterol Hepatol 2008;2(2):217–31.

49. Leclercq IA, Horsmans Y. Nonalcoholic fatty liver disease: the potential role of nutritional management. Curr Opin Clin Nutr Metab Care 2008;11(6):766–73.

50. Caldwell S, Lazo M. Is exercise an effective treatment for NASH? Knowns and unknowns. Ann Hepatol 2009;8(Suppl 1):S60–6.

51. Harrison SA, Fecht W, Brunt EM, et al. Orlistat for overweight subjects with nonalcoholic steatohepatitis: a randomized, prospective trial. Hepatology 2009;49(1): 80–6.

52. Kral JG, Naslund E. Surgical treatment of obesity. Nat Clin Pract Endocrinol Metab 2007;3(8):574–83.

53. Hansen EN, Torquati A, Abumrad NN. Results of bariatric surgery. Annu Rev Nutr 2006;26:481–511.

54. Mummadi RR, Kasturi KS, Chennareddygari S, et al. Effect of bariatric surgery on nonalcoholic fatty liver disease: systematic review and meta-analysis. Clin Gastroenterol Hepatol 2008;6(12):1396–402.

55. Rafiq N, Younossi ZM. Effects of weight loss on nonalcoholic fatty liver disease. Semin Liver Dis 2008;28(4):427–33.

56. Mathurin P, Hollebecque A, Arnalsteen L, et al. Prospective study of the long-term effects of bariatric surgery on liver injury in patients without advanced disease. Gastroenterology 2009;137(2):532–40.

57. Trakhtenbroit MA, Leichman JG, Algahim MF, et al. Body weight, insulin resistance, and serum adipokine levels 2 years after 2 types of bariatric surgery. Am J Med 2009;122(5):435–42.

58. Vuppalanchi R, Chalasani N. Nonalcoholic fatty liver disease and nonalcoholic steatohepatitis: selected practical issues in their evaluation and management. Hepatology 2009;49(1):306–17.

59. Browning JD. Statins and hepatic steatosis: perspectives from the Dallas Heart Study. Hepatology 2006;44(2):466–71.

60. Kiyici M, Gulten M, Gurel S, et al. Ursodeoxycholic acid and atorvastatin in the treatment of nonalcoholic steatohepatitis. Can J Gastroenterol 2003;17(12):713–8.

61. Hyogo H, Tazuma S, Arihiro K, et al. Efficacy of atorvastatin for the treatment of nonalcoholic steatohepatitis with dyslipidemia. Metabolism 2008;57(12):1711–8.
62. Laurin J, Lindor KD, Crippin JS, et al. Ursodeoxycholic acid or clofibrate in the treatment of non-alcohol-induced steatohepatitis: a pilot study. Hepatology 1996;23(6):1464–7.
63. Yokohama S, Yoneda M, Haneda M, et al. Therapeutic efficacy of an angiotensin II receptor antagonist in patients with nonalcoholic steatohepatitis. Hepatology 2004;40(5):1222–5.
64. Lavine JE. Vitamin E treatment of nonalcoholic steatohepatitis in children: a pilot study. J Pediatr 2000;136(6):734–8.
65. Adams LA, Angulo P. Vitamins E and C for the treatment of NASH: duplication of results but lack of demonstration of efficacy. Am J Gastroenterol 2003;98(11): 2348–50.
66. Harrison SA, Torgerson S, Hayashi P, et al. Vitamin E and vitamin C treatment improves fibrosis in patients with nonalcoholic steatohepatitis. Am J Gastroenterol 2003;98(11):2485–90.
67. Yakaryilmaz F, Guliter S, Savas B, et al. Effects of vitamin E treatment on peroxisome proliferator-activated receptor-alpha expression and insulin resistance in patients with non-alcoholic steatohepatitis: results of a pilot study. Intern Med J 2007;37(4):229–35.
68. Abdelmalek MF, Angulo P, Jorgensen RA, et al. Betaine, a promising new agent for patients with nonalcoholic steatohepatitis: results of a pilot study. Am J Gastroenterol 2001;96(9):2711–7.
69. Abdelmalek MF, Sanderson SO, Angulo P, et al. Betaine for nonalcoholic fatty liver disease: results of a randomized placebo-controlled trial. Hepatology 2009;50(6): 1818–26.
70. Georgescu EF, Georgescu M. Therapeutic options in non-alcoholic steatohepatitis (NASH). Are all agents alike? Results of a preliminary study. J Gastrointestin Liver Dis 2007;16(1):39–46.
71. Nair S, Diehl AM, Wiseman M, et al. Metformin in the treatment of non-alcoholic steatohepatitis: a pilot open label trial. Aliment Pharmacol Ther 2004;20(1):23–8.
72. Marchesini G, Brizi M, Bianchi G, et al. Metformin in non-alcoholic steatohepatitis. Lancet 2001;358(9285):893–4.
73. Bugianesi E, Gentilcore E, Manini R, et al. A randomized controlled trial of metformin versus vitamin E or prescriptive diet in nonalcoholic fatty liver disease. Am J Gastroenterol 2005;100(5):1082–90.
74. Lindor KD, Kowdley KV, Heathcote EJ, et al. Ursodeoxycholic acid for treatment of nonalcoholic steatohepatitis: results of a randomized trial. Hepatology 2004; 39(3):770–8.
75. Chamulitrat W, Burhenne J, Rehlen T, et al. Bile salt-phospholipid conjugate ursodeoxycholyl lysophosphatidylethanolamide as a hepatoprotective agent. Hepatology 2009;50(1):143–54.
76. Dufour JF, Oneta CM, Gonvers JJ, et al. Randomized placebo-controlled trial of ursodeoxycholic acid with vitamin e in nonalcoholic steatohepatitis. Clin Gastroenterol Hepatol 2006;4(12):1537–43.
77. Loguercio C, Federico A, Tuccillo C, et al. Beneficial effects of a probiotic VSL#3 on parameters of liver dysfunction in chronic liver diseases. J Clin Gastroenterol 2005;39(6):540–3.
78. Lirussi F, Mastropasqua E, Orando S, et al. Probiotics for non-alcoholic fatty liver disease and/or steatohepatitis. Cochrane Database Syst Rev 2007;(1): CD005165.

79. Flier JS, Maekalanos JJA. Gut check: testing a role for the intestinal microbiome in human obesity. Sci Transl Med 2009;1(6):1–3.
80. Witek RP, Stone WC, Karaca FG, et al. Pan-caspase inhibitor VX-166 reduces fibrosis in an animal model of nonalcoholic steatohepatitis. Hepatology 2009; 50(5):1421–30.
81. Feldstein AE, Canbay A, Angulo P, et al. Hepatocyte apoptosis and fas expression are prominent features of human nonalcoholic steatohepatitis. Gastroenterology 2003;125(2):437–43.
82. Mallat A, Lotersztajn S. Cannabinoid receptors as therapeutic targets in the management of liver diseases. Drug News Perspect 2008;21(7):363–8.
83. Chaudhary N, Pfluger PT. Metabolic benefits from Sirt1 and Sirt1 activators. Curr Opin Clin Nutr Metab Care 2009;12(4):431–7.
84. Marchesini G, Brizi M, Morselli-Labate AM, et al. Association of nonalcoholic fatty liver disease with insulin resistance. Am J Med 1999;107(5):450–5.
85. Caldwell SH, Hespenheide EE, Redick JA, et al. A pilot study of a thiazolidinedione, troglitazone, in nonalcoholic steatohepatitis. Am J Gastroenterol 2001; 96(2):519–25.
86. Neuschwander-Tetri BA, Brunt EM, Wehmeier KR, et al. Improved nonalcoholic steatohepatitis after 48 weeks of treatment with the PPAR-gamma ligand rosiglitazone. Hepatology 2003;38(4):1008–17.
87. Sanyal AJ, Mofrad PS, Contos MJ, et al. A pilot study of vitamin E versus vitamin E and pioglitazone for the treatment of nonalcoholic steatohepatitis. Clin Gastroenterol Hepatol 2004;2(12):1107–15.
88. Ratziu V, Giral P, Jacqueminet S, et al. Rosiglitazone for nonalcoholic steatohepatitis: one-year results of the randomized placebo-controlled Fatty Liver Improvement with Rosiglitazone Therapy (FLIRT) Trial. Gastroenterology 2008;135(1): 100–10.
89. Ratziu V, Charlotte F, Bernhardt C, et al. Long-term efficacy of rosiglitazone in nonalcoholic steatohepatitis: results of the fatty liver improvement by rosiglitazone therapy (FLIRT 2) extension trial. Hepatology 2009. [Epub ahead of print].
90. Yki-Jarvinen H. Thiazolidinediones and the liver in humans. Curr Opin Lipidol 2009;20(6):477–83.

Pharmacologic Therapies for Obesity

Lee M. Kaplan, MD, PhD

KEYWORDS

- Obesity treatment • Pharmacology treatments obesity
- Weight loss medication

The development of effective pharmacologic therapies has been both the greatest hope and one of the greatest disappointments in the field of obesity. At its root, obesity is a complex metabolic and behavioral disorder that disrupts normal body weight regulatory mechanisms. Logically, both the metabolic and behavioral components of body weight regulation should be amenable to pharmacologic treatment, and several agents have been developed that influence eating behavior, food intake, nutrient absorption, and energy expenditure.[1] These medications induce weight loss, but to a lesser extent and for a shorter period than would be considered ideal by either patients or physicians. Moreover, many of these agents have been associated with unacceptable adverse effects, in many cases as a direct result of their therapeutic mechanism of action. These side effects, including the euphoric and addictive effects of amphetamines, the hypertensive and arrhythmogenic effects of the adrenergic agents, the cardiac valvular effects of fenfluramine, and the steatorrhea associated with orlistat, have significantly curtailed the use of these drugs and, in some cases, required their complete withdrawal from the market.

Recent studies of the physiology of body weight regulation have demonstrated the complexity of this control system and have identified numerous novel targets for therapeutic intervention.[2] These studies provide hope that new, more specific agents will provide more effective and durable treatment of obesity with fewer side effects. The very complexity of weight regulation, however, and the powerful systems to defend against real or perceived starvation, makes it unlikely that a single pathway, cell, or molecule will prove to be the Achilles heel of obesity. Thus, long-term effective treatment is likely to require a multimodal approach, with multiple drugs aimed at different targets or novel combinations of specific pharmacologic, nutritional, endoscopic, and surgical approaches.

Currently available pharmacologic therapies for obesity can be effective adjuncts to diet- and exercise-based behavioral therapies, typically increasing the amount of

This work was supported by grants DK088661, LM008748, and DK046200 from the National Institutes of Health.
MGH Weight Center and Gastrointestinal Unit, Massachusetts General Hospital and Harvard Medical School, 50 Staniford Street, 4th Floor, Boston, MA 02114, USA
E-mail address: LMKaplan@partners.org

weight loss by 4% to 6% over 1 to 2 years (eg, from a weight loss of 4% to a weight loss of 8% during this time).[3,4] In nearly all cases, however, the maximal effect appears to occur within the first year of therapy (often within the first 6 months) with partial regain of lost weight thereafter. In addition, the response to each medication varies widely from patient to patient, with a small number of patients (typically 2%–5%) exhibiting considerably more weight loss than average, and a significant portion experiencing no weight loss.

For the currently available weight loss medications (regardless of the mechanism of action), the criterion of a 4-pound weight loss in 4 weeks is a helpful guideline. Weight loss of lesser magnitude provides good evidence that the medication has little therapeutic value for the patient. Given the potential for adverse effects, such modest weight loss is a strong indication for stopping the drug. For patients who lose 4 or more pounds in the first month, it is not clear how much additional weight loss should occur for the drug to be continued. Many physicians require that patients lose 4 pounds per month for a minimum of 3 months (12 pounds total) to consider the medication clinically effective. Thereafter, if a patient maintains the lower weight, the drug is still considered effective, since it is preventing the weight regain that occurs in more than 90% of patients upon cessation of treatment. For each of these drugs, human and animal studies suggest that they work less by causing weight loss per se than by causing the patient (or animal) to seek a specific, lower weight. For each drug and for each patient, there appears to be a maximum achievable weight loss. Continuing the drug is usually necessary to maintain all or most of the lost weight, and cessation is almost always associated with rapid regain of the lost weight.[5,6]

Weight loss medications are usually reserved for patients who have failed more standard behavioral interventions, including various combinations of diet- and exercise-based approaches. **Box 1** shows the standard criteria for use of these agents.[7]

MEDICATIONS APPROVED FOR THE TREATMENT OF OBESITY

Table 1 lists the medications most commonly used for the treatment of obesity. These drugs are specifically approved by the US Food and Drug Administration (FDA) for this indication. **Table 2** lists medications approved for other indications that have been found in one or more clinical studies to generate a significant weight loss effect. Three drugs, diethylpropion, phendimetrazine, and benzphetamine, are approved by the FDA but classified as Schedule III drugs by the Drug Enforcement Administration because of their high potential for abuse. These drugs have little or no role in the routine management of obesity and are not considered further here.

Box 1
Clinical criteria for pharmacologic therapy for obesity

Body mass index (BMI)>30 kg/m² or BMI>27 kg/m² in association with significant medical complications

Failure of behavioral approaches, including diet and exercise regimens

No strong contraindications to the medication used

For continued treatment, weight loss of ≥4 pounds per month for each of the first three months

Table 1
Medications approved by the FDA specifically for weight loss indication[a]

Medication	Typical Dosing	Classification	Common Adverse Effects
Phentermine[4,a]	15–37.5 mg/d	Adrenergic agent	Tachycardia, hypertension
Sibutramine[4,8,a,b]	10-15 mg/d	Serotonergic or adrenergic	Hypertension, tachycardia
Orlistat[4,8]	120 mg tid	Lipase inhibitor	Malabsorption, steatorrhea

[a] Phentermine is approved by the FDA for 3 months' use and sibutramine and orlistat are each approved for one year's use. Use in clinical practice varies widely.
[b] Use of sibutramine in patients taking serotonin-selective reuptake inhibitors (SSRI) is relatively contraindicated because of the risk of serotonin syndrome.

PHENTERMINE

Phentermine is an adrenergic reuptake inhibitor that augments adrenergic signaling in the brain and peripheral tissues. It is therefore thought to promote weight loss by activation of the sympathetic nervous system with resulting decrease in food intake and increased resting energy expenditure.[14,15]

Phentermine is the safe half of the phentermine-fenfluramine (phen-fen) combination therapy introduced in the 1990s. Unlike fenfluramine, phentermine has no known effects on cardiac valves.[16–18] As a adrenergic agonist, however, it can be associated with tachycardia and, less commonly, hypertension.[3] Thus, phentermine should be used with caution in people at significant risk for hemodynamic or cardiovascular complications of tachycardia and those with uncontrolled hypertension. It is good practice to monitor the pulse and blood pressure of patients closely during the first few weeks of phentermine therapy.

Because phentermine is no longer covered by patent protection and there are several proprietary and generic formulations available, it is the least expensive and most commonly prescribed medication for weight loss.[19] It comes in two major forms, phentermine resin (Ionamin) and phentermine-HCl. Normal dosing is 15 to 30mg/d for phentermine resin and 18.75 to 37.5mg/d for phentermine-HCl. An acceptable therapeutic response is considered as 4 pounds per 4 weeks for at least the first 8 to

Table 2
Medications approved by the FDA for other indications that exhibit weight loss promoting effects

Medication	Typical Dosing[a]	Primary Indications	Common Adverse Effects
Bupropion[9,b]	150-300 mg/d	Depression	Anticholinergic, agitation
Metformin[10]	500-1000 mg/d	Type 2 diabetes	Hepatic oxidative injury
Exenatide[11]	5–10 mcg bid	Type 2 diabetes	Nausea
Topiramate[12]	50-100 mg/d	Seizure disorder Migraine headaches	Cognitive impairment, peripheral neuropathy
Zonisamide[13]	400-600 mg/d	Seizure disorder	Cognitive impairment

These agents are typically approved for life-long use for their specific indication.
[a] Typical dosing for use as a weight loss agent. Dosing for primary indication may be higher.
[b] Use of phentermine, sibutramine or bupropion in patients taking monoamine oxidase (MAO) inhibitors is strongly contraindicated because of the risk of severe cardiovascular events. Bupropion is contraindicated in patients with bipolar disease.

12 weeks of therapy, when given with or without associated dietary and exercise counseling.

Although approved by the FDA for only 3 months' use, many experts advocate longer-term use in patients who demonstrate a good therapeutic response during the first 3 months. As with other weight loss medications, the weight loss generally stops within 3 to 6 months of initiation. For patients who have lost a significant amount of weight during this time, continuation of the drug is nonetheless valuable to prevent weight regain.

SIBUTRAMINE

Sibutramine, a monoamine reuptake inhibitor, enhances adrenergic, serotonergic and dopaminergic signaling in the brain. Thus, it has pharmacologic characteristics that are similar to, if weaker than, those of phen-fen. Unlike fenfluramine, which has been withdrawn because of the risk of carcinoid-like cardiac valvular disease, sibutramine's serotonergic effects have not been associated with valvular abnormalities.

Sibutramine treatment is associated with an average weight loss of approximately 5% to 8%, as compared with 2% to 4% in participants receiving placebo.[6,8,20] Most of the randomized, controlled trials include dietary or exercise counseling for participants in both the treatment and placebo groups, which likely accounts for the weight loss in the placebo group. Thus, sibutramine itself appears to be associated with an average weight loss of approximately 3% to 4% during the first 6 to 12 months of treatment. Extension of therapy for up to 2 years is associated with an average regain of approximately half of the weight lost initially. However, in one large trial, of the participants who experienced greater than or equal to 5% weight loss on sibutramine, more than 25% maintained the full weight loss when sibutramine treatment was continued for an additional year. As with other therapies for obesity, there is a wide patient-to-patient variation in response. A small percentage of patients exhibits dramatic weight loss, and a significant number experience no weight loss benefit at all. To date, no clinically relevant predictors of outcome after sibutramine or other weight loss medications have been identified.[3,6,8,15,20]

The normal dosing for sibutramine in adults is 10 to 15 mg/d taken once daily. Many physicians prefer to start with 10 mg/d and increase to 15 mg/d as clinically required. Doses higher than 15 mg/d have not been demonstrated to have increased efficacy, and they are associated with a greater risk of side effects. Patients who lose greater than or equal to 4 lb/mo for at least 3 months are considered clinical responders and are good candidates for continuation of this treatment. As with other pharmacologic therapies, weight loss generally stops after approximately 3 to 6 months. Nonetheless, for patients who have lost a significant amount of weight by this time, continuing treatment appears to decrease the rate and magnitude of weight regain. Sibutramine is currently approved by the FDA for up to 1 year of treatment. However, many specialists use it in clinical responders for as long as it appears effective in preventing weight regain.

In most patients, the major side effects of sibutramine relate to its adrenergic properties. Approximately 10% to 15% of patients experience hypertension that can be managed by antihypertensive therapy or discontinuing the sibutramine; fewer than 3% of patients need to discontinue this drug because of uncontrolled hypertension. Patients with preexisting hypertension undergoing sibutramine therapy need to be monitored closely for exacerbation of their hypertension and their antihypertensive regimen adjusted as required. A small number of patients exhibit tachycardia with sibutramine, and this drug should be avoided in patients who are at elevated risk for life-threatening tachyarrhythmias and those who are unlikely to tolerate tachycardia of any cause. Other, generally less severe and dangerous side effects include anticholinergic-like effects.[8,14,15]

Use of sibutramine in patients taking serotonin-selective reuptake inhibitors (SSRIs) is relatively contraindicated because of an increased risk of serotonin syndrome, which is marked by some combination of flushing, diarrhea, and hypotension. As a result, sibutramine should only be prescribed to patients on SSRIs when both agents are strongly indicated and the patient is closely supervised by a physician well versed in the use of these agents alone and in combination.

ORLISTAT

Orlistat (Xenical, Alli), an inhibitor of pancreatic and intestinal lipases present in the intestinal lumen, prevents the breakdown of ingested triglycerides into absorbable fatty acids and monoacylglycerols.[8,14] When taken with meals, orlistat is capable of inhibiting the absorption of up to 30% of ingested fat. Clinical trials have revealed that orlistat treatment (120 mg three times a day with meals) in the setting of nutritional counseling is associated with a weight loss of approximately 9% at 1 year. Subjects receiving a placebo along with the counseling lost nearly 6%, suggesting that orlistat itself is responsible for approximately 3% body weight loss on average.[4,8,15,21] In one study, extension of orlistat therapy to 2 years is associated with a regain of approximately one-third of the initial weight loss, versus two-thirds regain in those who took placebo during the second year. Some clinicians preferentially prescribe orlistat to patients who consume a high-fat diet; there is no evidence, however, that such patients respond better to this agent. Moreover, although conceptually attractive, there is no good evidence that the diminishing effects of orlistat in the second year of treatment results from substitution of carbohydrates for fats in the patients' diets. Some patients decrease their intake of fats to limit the gastrointestinal side effects of the drug, but the efficacy of this strategy is not clear. As with other weight loss medications, the magnitude of weight loss on orlistat is somewhat less in patients with type 2 diabetes mellitus.[22]

As seen with other therapies, weight loss from orlistat treatment is associated with improvements in several comorbidities of obesity, including blood pressure, insulin resistance, and serum lipid levels. Use of orlistat has been limited by its limited efficacy and the high rate of gastrointestinal side effects. These side effects include flatulence, steatorrhea, increased stool frequency, fecal incontinence, and oily rectal discharge. The associated malabsorption can lead to deficiencies of the fat-soluble vitamins A, D, E, and K, and all patients on orlistat should receive a daily supplement enriched for these vitamins, given at least 2 hours before or after each orlistat dose.[8,21] Because of the higher rate of vitamin D deficiency in people with obesity and the associated risk of metabolic bone disease, vitamin D levels should be measured before starting orlistat and periodically (eg, every six months) during therapy, with supplementation to achieve a serum 1,25-OH-vitamin D level of greater than or equal to 30 IU/mL.

NOVEL PHARMACOLOGIC THERAPIES

Several new pharmacologic therapies have recently been examined in late-stage clinical trials. They include lorcaserin, a combination of naltrexone and bupropion, and a combination of phentermine and topiramate. Each of these agents has been demonstrated to induce significant weight loss in patients who are overweight or have obesity.

Lorcaserin

Lorcaserin is a selective agonist of the 5-HT$_{2C}$ serotonin receptor. Signaling through the 5-HT$_{2C}$ receptor appears to be the primary mechanism by which serotonergic agents such as fenfluramine exert their weight loss-promoting effects. At clinically effective doses, lorcaserin does not activate the 5-HT$_{2B}$ receptor, which appears to be the receptor primarily responsible for the cardiac valvular disease associated with fenfluramine. Recent large, phase 3 trials of lorcaserin revealed no valvulopathy resulting from the use of this agent. These trials demonstrated an average 3.5% weight loss beyond that seen with placebo therapy.[2,23–26] As with other medications, there was a broad range of responses with a small but significant portion of patients experiencing considerable weight loss. For these patients, treatment with this medication is likely to be an effective strategy for long-term management of obesity. In addition, lorcaserin's good safety profile makes it an attractive agent for use in combination therapies. Its shared mechanism of action with fenfluramine suggests that a lorcaserin-phentermine combination therapy may be particularly effective. It is difficult to predict adverse effects of drug combinations; however, if lorcaserin is approved by the FDA, controlled studies will need to be done before such combinations are considered for routine clinical use.

Naltrexone-bupropion

Naltrexone is an opioid receptor antagonist that has been used as an adjunctive therapy for the treatment of substance abuse and addiction.[27] Although it does not induce substantial weight loss as a single agent, its effects on central weight regulatory mechanisms suggest that it could enhance the weight loss induced by other centrally acting agents. Bupropion has been shown to have modest but significant weight loss promoting effects. The combination of naltrexone and bupropion has recently been examined in a large phase 3 trial for the treatment of obesity. This study demonstrated that 1 year of treatment with this two-drug combination induced an approximate 4% weight loss beyond that seen with placebo therapy, similar to that seen with other pharmacologic therapies.[27–30] Because of the distinct mechanism of action of these two medications, naltrexone-bupropion may prove to be an attractive option for patients who are resistant to other agents.

Phentermine-topiramate

Several clinicians have noted that the combination of phentermine and topiramate can generate substantial weight loss in at least a subset of patients who exhibit little weight loss when treated with phentermine alone. These observations led to the development of fixed dose combinations of phentermine and topiramate.[12,31] A large, phase 3 clinical trial has shown that 1 year of treatment with this combination led to weight loss of up to 9% beyond that seen with placebo therapy. This degree of weight loss appears to be somewhat greater than that seen with the other medications currently approved by the FDA or in late stage clinical development. There have been no-head-to-head comparisons, however, and further studies will be needed to determine the relative effectiveness of these various treatments.[2,26,32–34] It is noteworthy that the doses of each agent used in the phentermine-topiramate combination studied were lower than the typical doses used for monotherapy with each drug. The ability to use lower doses of component drugs in combination therapies underscores the potential synergistic efficacy and improved benefit-risk profiles of drug combinations.

DISCREDITED MEDICATIONS
Fenfluramine

Fenfluramine and its biologically active enantiomer, dexfenfluramine, are monoamine secretagogues. They act by making more serotonin available at serotonergic synapses, and one effect of this increased synaptic serotonin is to diminish appetite and promote energy expenditure. The combination of fenfluramine and phentermine, an adrenergic agonist, was shown in the early 1990s to have dramatically improved effects (both numbers of positive responders and degree of weight loss) over either phentermine or fenfluramine alone.[34] Widespread use of this combination began in 1995 and was accelerated by FDA approval of dexfenfluramine (Redux) for weight loss in 1996. However, in 1997, a high rate of cardiac valvular abnormalities, most notably fibrosis reminiscent of carcinoid- or serotonin-associated heart disease, was seen in patients taking these agents.[16] Further epidemiologic examination linked these abnormalities with the fenfluramine, which was withdrawn from the market. Phentermine is still in widespread use for obesity treatment. It has none of the valvular effects associated with fenfluramine. In the years since fenfluramine was withdrawn, the risk of associated valvular disorders has been reevaluated and, while still significant, was found to be substantially lower than originally thought. Fortunately, many patients who exhibited valvular abnormalities from this medication have experienced partial or complete regression of these changes after the drug was discontinued.[17,18]

Ephedrine and Phenylpropanolamine

These agents had been sold as over-the-counter weight loss remedies until they were withdrawn in 2002 and 2004, respectively, after the FDA determined that they were unsafe for routine use.[35,36] Despite their widespread use in dietary supplements and herbal formulations, there have been few studies of their short- or long-term effectiveness in promoting weight loss. These agents have been associated with an increased risk of cardiovascular complications, including strokes and life-threatening arrhythmias, which led to the FDA recommendations that they be withdrawn. Current formulations of dietary supplements and other over-the-counter weight loss therapies sold in the United States do not include these compounds.

PHARMACOLOGIC TREATMENT OF DRUG-INDUCED WEIGHT GAIN

Many medications are associated with weight gain, including steroid hormones, thiazolidinediones, insulinotropic agents, and several classes of psychotropic drugs (**Box 2**). Treatment for drug-induced obesity is similar to that for "essential" obesity, with a heavy reliance on behavioral therapies to improve diet and increase physical activity. In some cases, however, drug-induced obesity may be more amenable to pharmacotherapy than other weight disorders. Weight gain associated with treatment of diabetes may be ameliorated or reversed by inclusion of metformin in the antidiabetic regimen, either in lieu of or in addition to thiazolidinediones or sulfonylureas. Whereas insulin, sulfonylureas, and thiazolidinediones promote weight gain and central fat redistribution, metformin often promotes weight loss. In the absence of associated weight loss, metformin tends to be weight-neutral, and substitution of other antidiabetic agents with metformin often results in modest weight loss. For patients with seizure or mood disorders in whom pharmacologic treatment has been associated with significant weight gain, topiramate and zonisamide may be particularly helpful.[12,22,37] Both of these agents are approved by the FDA for treatment of seizure disorders, and topiramate is also approved for the treatment of migraine headaches. In addition, they have been found to have mood stabilizing properties, making them reasonable alternatives to weight-promoting antidepressants and mood stabilizers such as olanzapine and clozapine.[37] In some cases of seizure and mood disorders, it is possible to change from these medications to ones that have fewer weight-promoting effects, including topiramate and zonisamide. Alternatively,

---

Box 2
Medications associated with weight gain

Steroid hormones

    Glucocorticoids

    Progesterone

Neurotropic and psychotropic medications

    Olanzapine (Zyprexa); clozapine (Clozaril)

    Valproic acid (Depakote)

    Lithium

    Phenothiazines

    Antidepressants: SSRIs, tricyclics, monoamine oxidase inhibitors

Diabetes treatments

    Sulfonylureas

    Insulin

    Thiazolidinediones (Actos, Avandia)

---

these weight loss-promoting mood stabilizers and anticonvulsants are often effective when added to the patient's regimen. Different practitioners follow widely different practice patterns relating to these medications. Where equivalent efficacy can be achieved with agents that inhibit further weight gain or promote reversal of previous obesity, this approach is generally accepted.

MEDICATION USE AFTER WEIGHT LOSS SURGERY

Although gastrointestinal weight loss surgery is a highly effective therapy for severe obesity, its efficacy varies considerably among individual patients. After Roux-en-Y gastric bypass, patients lose an average of 65% to 70% of their excess body weight within the first 1 to 2 years after surgery and maintain the loss of 50% to 55% of their excess body weight over more than 10 years.[38] Hatoum and colleagues have observed, however, that weight loss in individual patients varies from 20 to 120% of excess body weight at one year.[39] For many patients at the lower end of the weight loss distribution, the results of surgery are disappointing. Some clinicians have used medications in an attempt to enhance weight loss after surgery. No formal trials of this approach have yet been reported, but the centrally acting agents, including phentermine, sibutramine, and topiramate are attractive because of their ability to curb appetite in many patients. Orlistat in this setting appears inadvisable since it can exacerbate deficiencies of fat-soluble vitamins already depleted by the surgery itself. Prescribing any weight loss medication after surgery should be viewed as experimental, however, and should generally be limited to controlled trials by clinicians experienced in obesity treatment.

FUTURE CONSIDERATIONS

The increasing understanding of the normal mechanisms of weight regulation has given rise to numerous targets for new pharmacologic therapies and more than 80 drugs are now under active development for the treatment of obesity. Many of these agents are more narrowly directed than currently available options. Thus, there is hope that they will have a better adverse effect profile. Because the normal weight regulatory mechanisms are complex, and redundant systems are likely to be present to guard against starvation, it is unlikely that any single agent will be the holy grail of obesity therapy. Effective long-term control of weight by pharmacologic therapies will likely require multiple agents used in combination. The large number of drugs under development suggests that several moderately effective agents will emerge. Combinations of different moderately effective agents or combination of these agents with other therapies (eg, behavior modification, dietary manipulation, intestinal infusions, electrical stimulation, or endoscopic or laparoscopic surgery) will likely generate the greatest sustainable weight loss. Design of some of these combinations will be guided by our advancing knowledge about the physiologic effects of weight loss surgery and the mechanisms used by this very effective treatment to effect durable weight loss. The identification of increasingly safe and moderately effective medications for obesity will likely be the basis for new and very effective combination approaches, even if they have limited utility as single agents. Such combinations will likely provide the greatest opportunity for the effective nonsurgical treatment of obesity.

REFERENCES

1. Bray GA. Medications for weight reduction. Endocrinol Metab Clin North Am 2008;37:923–42.
2. Chakrabarti R. Pharmacotherapy of obesity: emerging drugs and targets. Expert Opin Ther Targets 2009;13:195–207.
3. Bray GA. Lifestyle and pharmacological approaches to weight loss: efficacy and safety. J Clin Endocrinol Metab 2008;93:S81–8.
4. Padwal R, Li SK, Lau DC. Long-term pharmacotherapy for overweight and obesity: a systematic review and meta-analysis of randomized controlled trials. Int J Obes Relat Metab Disord 2003;27:1437–46.
5. Bray GA, Greenway FL. Pharmacological treatment of the overweight patient. Pharmacol Rev 2007;59:151–84.
6. Padwal R, Li SK, Lau DC. Long-term pharmacotherapy for obesity and overweight. Cochrane Database Syst Rev 2003;CD004094.
7. Clinical guidelines on the identification, evaluation, and treatment of overweight and obesity in adults—the evidence report. National Institutes of Health. Obes Res 1998;6(Suppl 2):51S–209S.
8. Leung WY, Thomas GN, Chan JC, et al. Weight management and current options in pharmacotherapy: orlistat and sibutramine. Clin Ther 2003;25:58–80.
9. Jain AK, Kaplan RA, Gadde KM, et al. Bupropion SR vs. placebo for weight loss in obese patients with depressive symptoms. Obes Res 2002;10:1049–56.
10. Harborne LR, Sattar N, Norman JE, et al. Metformin and weight loss in obese women with polycystic ovary syndrome: comparison of doses. J Clin Endocrinol Metab 2005;90:4593–8.
11. Mafong DD, Henry RR. Exenatide as a treatment for diabetes and obesity: implications for cardiovascular risk reduction. Curr Atheroscler Rep 2008;10:55–60.
12. Astrup A, Toubro S. Topiramate: a new potential pharmacological treatment for obesity. Obes Res 2004;12(Suppl):167S–73S.
13. Gadde KM, Franciscy DM, Wagner HR 2nd, et al. Zonisamide for weight loss in obese adults: a randomized controlled trial. JAMA 2003;289:1820–5.
14. Bray GA, Ryan DH. Drug treatment of the overweight patient. Gastroenterology 2007;132:2239–52.

15. Neovius M, Johansson K, Rossner S. Head-to-head studies evaluating efficacy of pharmaco-therapy for obesity: a systematic review and meta-analysis. Obes Rev 2008;9:420–7.
16. Connolly HM, Crary JL, McGoon MD, et al. Valvular heart disease associated with fenfluramine-phentermine. N Engl J Med 1997;337:581–8.
17. Dahl CF, Allen MR. Regression and progression of valvulopathy associated with fenfluramine and phentermine. Ann Intern Med 2002;136:489.
18. Volmar KE, Hutchins GM. Aortic and mitral fenfluramine-phentermine valvulopathy in 64 patients treated with anorectic agents. Arch Pathol Lab Med 2001; 125:1555–61.
19. Neovius M, Narbro K. Cost-effectiveness of pharmacological anti-obesity treatments: a systematic review. Int J Obes (Lond) 2008;32:1752–63.
20. Wadden TA, Berkowitz RI, Womble LG, et al. Randomized trial of lifestyle modification and pharmacotherapy for obesity. N Engl J Med 2005;353:2111–20.
21. Bray GA. Are non-prescription medications needed for weight control? Obesity (Silver Spring) 2008;16:509–14.
22. Eliasson B, Gudbjornsdottir S, Cederholm J, et al. Weight loss and metabolic effects of topiramate in overweight and obese type 2 diabetic patients: randomized double-blind placebo-controlled trial. Int J Obes (Lond) 2007;31:1140–7.
23. Smith SR, Aronne LJ, Burns CM, et al. Sustained weight loss following 12-month pramlintide treatment as an adjunct to lifestyle intervention in obesity. Diabetes Care 2008;31:1816–23.
24. Idelevich E, Kirch W, Schindler C. Current pharmacotherapeutic concepts for the treatment of obesity in adults. Ther Adv Cardiovasc Dis 2009;3:75–90.
25. Jeon MK, Cheon HG. Promising strategies for obesity pharmacotherapy: melanocortin-4 (MC-4) receptor agonists and melanin concentrating hormone (MCH) receptor-1 antagonists. Curr Top Med Chem 2009;9:504–38.
26. Mayer MA, Hocht C, Puyo A, et al. Recent advances in obesity pharmacotherapy. Curr Clin Pharmacol 2009;4:53–61.
27. Lee MW, Fujioka K. Naltrexone for the treatment of obesity: review and update. Expert Opin Pharmacother 2009;10:1841–5.
28. Greenway FL, Dunayevich E, Tollefson G, et al. Comparison of combined bupropion and naltrexone therapy for obesity with monotherapy and placebo. J Clin Endocrinol Metab 2009;94:4898–906.
29. Padwal R. Contrave, a bupropion and naltrexone combination therapy for the potential treatment of obesity. Curr Opin Investig Drugs 2009;10:1117–25.
30. Plodkowski RA, Nguyen Q, Sundaram U, et al. Bupropion and naltrexone: a review of their use individually and in combination for the treatment of obesity. Expert Opin Pharmacother 2009;10:1069–81.
31. Klonoff DC, Greenway F. Drugs in the pipeline for the obesity market. J Diabetes Sci Technol 2008;2:913–8.
32. Gadde KM, Allison DB. Combination therapy for obesity and metabolic disease. Curr Opin Endocrinol Diabetes Obes 2009;16:353–8.
33. Isidro ML, Cordido F. Drug treatment of obesity: established and emerging therapies. Mini Rev Med Chem 2009;9:664–73.
34. Weintraub M, Sundaresan PR, Schuster B, et al. Long-term weight control study. IV (weeks 156 to 190). The second double-blind phase. Clin Pharmacol Ther 1992;51:608–14.
35. Drug Enforcement Administration (DEA), Justice. Implementation of the comprehensive methamphetamine control of 1996; regulation of pseudoephedrine, phenylpropanolamine, and combination ephedrine drug products and reports

of certain transactions to nonregulated persons. Final rule. Fed Regist 2002;67: 14853–62.

36. Food and Drug Administration, HHS. Final rule declaring dietary supplements containing ephedrine alkaloids adulterated because they present an unreasonable risk. Final rule. Fed Regist 2004;69:6787–854.

37. Shank RP, Maryanoff BE. Molecular pharmacodynamics, clinical therapeutics, and pharmacokinetics of topiramate. CNS Neurosci Ther 2008;14:120–42.

38. Buchwald H, Avidor Y, Braunwald E, et al. Bariatric surgery: a systematic review and meta-analysis. JAMA 2004;292:1724–37.

39. Hatoum IJ, Stein HK, Merrifield BF, et al. Capacity for physical activity predicts weight loss after Roux-en-Y gastric bypass. Obesity (Silver Spring) 2009;17:92–9.

Preoperative Gastrointestinal Assessment Before Bariatric Surgery

David Greenwald, MD[a,b,*]

KEYWORDS

- Obesity • Gastrointestinal tract • Bariatric surgery
- Endoscopy

Obesity is a major health problem throughout the world, and nearly one-third of the population of the United States is considered obese.[1] Obesity surgery is frequently considered among the treatment options for the severely overweight, and surgically induced weight loss has become the best treatment for many morbidly obese people. Before bariatric surgery, an extensive preoperative assessment is warranted to evaluate whether a patient is appropriate for a given operation and to clarify factors that may affect the outcome of a planned procedure. Gastroenterologists often are called in for the preoperative gastrointestinal (GI) assessment of a patient who is being considered for bariatric surgery. This article explores some of the relevant issues for gastroenterologists to consider when consulting on these patients.

PREOPERATIVE EVALUATION

Patients who are candidates for bariatric surgery are evaluated in the same fashion, regardless of the type of bariatric procedure that is being considered. Evaluation typically includes a thorough assessment of the indications for surgically induced weight loss, identification of factors that may mitigate the success of a procedure, and a search for comorbid disease. Typical assessments include psychological testing, nutrition evaluation, and medical assessment.[2]

Nutritional Assessment

The gastroenterologist is a part of the multidisciplinary team, and so an understanding of the nutritional assessment of the patients who are preparing for bariatric surgery is

[a] Division of Gastroenterology, Montefiore Medical Center, 111 East 210th Street, Bronx, NY 10467, USA
[b] Albert Einstein College of Medicine, Bronx, NY, USA
* Division of Gastroenterology, Montefiore Medical Center, 111 East 210th Street, Bronx, NY 10467.
E-mail address: dgreenwa@montefiore.org

Gastroenterol Clin N Am 39 (2010) 81–86
doi:10.1016/j.gtc.2009.12.012
0889-8553/10/$ – see front matter © 2010 Elsevier Inc. All rights reserved.

important. In general, a nutritionist will provide a complete nutritional assessment and will coordinate preoperative weight loss attempts. Patients who lose at least 10% of their excess body weight preoperatively have more rapid loss of weight and shorter hospital stays after surgery.[3] The use of a very-low-calorie diet for 6 weeks before planned surgery is associated with an improved access to the stomach during laparoscopic surgery and a reduction in liver volume by 20%.[4,5]

Medical Assessment

The general medical assessment of a patient who is being considered for bariatric surgery is similar to that for any other major abdominal surgery (**Box 1**).[6,7] Patients are usually evaluated with laboratory testing that may include complete blood counts, metabolic profile, coagulation profile, ferritin level, thyroid function testing, and a lipid profile. For those in whom a malabsorptive procedure is being contemplated, vitamin B_{12} and fat-soluble vitamin levels may be considered. Pulmonary assessment often includes a chest radiograph, arterial blood gas measurement, and tests of pulmonary function. Cardiac assessment includes an electrocardiogram and may also include a stress test to identify unsuspected coronary artery disease. Sleep apnea is an important consideration in many obese patients, and so a sleep study may be part of the evaluation.

Box 1
Typical preoperative studies in patients undergoing bariatric surgery

Preoperative blood testing

    Complete blood count

    Metabolic profile

    Coagulation profile

    Ferritin

    Thyroid function test

    Lipid profile

    Vitamin B_{12}

    Fat-soluble vitamin levels

Cardiac

    Electrocardiogram

    Consider exercise stress test

Pulmonary

    Chest radiograph

    Arterial blood gas

    Pulmonary function testing

Sleep study

GI evaluation

    Upper GI series

    Upper endoscopy

    Abdominal ultrasonography

    Helicobacter pylori testing

GI Assessment

A thorough assessment of the GI tract before bariatric surgery is important to ensure successful outcomes. This assessment may include endoscopy, testing for *Helicobacter pylori*, and evaluation of the liver and gall bladder.

Upper endoscopy

The role of upper endoscopy in the preoperative evaluation of patients who are being considered for bariatric surgery is to detect upper GI abnormalities, even in asymptomatic patients.[8] Many patients with symptoms of dyspepsia, dysphagia, and reflux are evaluated with endoscopy, and the situation of an obese patient with these complaints is no different. Many studies have demonstrated that routine preoperative endoscopy in the bariatric patient detects various abnormalities that need specific approaches before surgery and that such preoperative endoscopy is warranted.[9] It is important to remember that some operations done for obesity, for example, Roux-en-Y gastrojejunal bypass (RYGB) and sleeve gastrectomy with duodenal switch and biliopancreatic diversion, make the distal stomach and duodenum inaccessible after the surgery. It would be reasonable to perform a preoperative examination of the upper GI tract is this setting.[8]

Endoscopy is useful in the preoperative assessment of the bariatric patient to find or treat lesions that might lead to alterations in the type of surgery that has been planned, that might cause complications in the patient postoperatively, or that might lead to symptoms after surgery. In one study, esophagogastroduodenoscopy before bariatric surgery identified abnormalities in nearly 90% of patients, with 62% having clinically important findings.[10] The most common lesions identified were hiatal hernia (40%), gastritis (29%), esophagitis (9%), gastric ulcer (4%), Barrett esophagus (3%), and esophageal ulcers (3%).[10] Another study of 626 patients detected abnormalities in 46% of the patients, including gastritis (21%), esophagitis (16%), hiatal hernia (11%), and duodenitis (8%). One case of gastric cancer was detected.[9] Another case report describes an early gastric cancer detected in the preoperative assessment for bariatric surgery.[11] Many other studies have demonstrated that routine endoscopy before laparoscopic adjustable gastric band,[12,13] vertical banded gastroplasty,[14] and Roux-en-Y procedures can identify many abnormalities. A recent meta-analysis demonstrated that obesity is associated with a significantly increased risk of gastroesophageal reflux disease, erosive esophagitis, and esophageal adenocarcinoma, making endoscopic evaluation warranted to detect such abnormalities preoperatively.[15] Two studies have demonstrated that findings of endoscopy led to a delay in surgery or a change in the surgical approach.[10,16] European Society guidelines recommend upper endoscopy in all patients as a part of the preassessment before bariatric surgery, whether or not the patient has symptoms.[17] Contrast studies, such as an upper GI series, may provide additional information to an endoscopy or may be an alternative; in one study of morbidly obese patients, radiographs were found to be superior to endoscopy in diagnosing sliding hiatal hernias before gastric bypass.[18,19]

Concern about the safety of sedation for endoscopy in the severely obese patient has led to investigation. In general, endoscopy is safe and effective in this population, although an increased risk of hypoxemia has been demonstrated in those with a body mass index greater than 28, and obesity may make rescue from complications of oversedation, such as mask ventilation, more difficult.[20] Madan and colleagues[21] found that monitored anesthesia care with propofol was equivalent to endoscopist-administered sedation with benzodiazepines and narcotics in a randomized trial of 100 morbidly obese patients who underwent upper endoscopy before bariatric surgery, although there was a trend toward some better outcomes with monitored anesthesia care.

An American Society for Gastrointestinal Endoscopy (ASGE) guideline, on the role of endoscopy in the bariatric surgery patient, published in 2008, has the following recommendations[8]:

1. An upper endoscopy should be performed in all patients with upper-GI tract symptoms who are to undergo bariatric surgery
2. Upper endoscopy should be considered in all patients who are to undergo an RYGB, regardless of the presence of symptoms
3. In patients without symptoms and who were undergoing gastric banding, a preoperative upper endoscopy should be considered to exclude large hernias that may change the surgical approach.

Evaluation and treatment of H pylori

Preoperative testing for H pylori has been advocated in patients having bariatric surgery. H pylori infection rates in this group are comparable to those seen in the general population, with H pylori reported to be present in 30% to 40% of the patients being considered for bariatric surgery. Noninvasive urease testing that was positive for H pylori was associated with the patient having an abnormal endoscopy more frequently than H pylori negative noninvasive urease testing (94% vs 51%).[22] Schirmer and colleagues[16] reported that patients tested for H pylori had a lower incidence of postoperative marginal ulcers (2.4%) than did patients who did not undergo such screening (6.8%). If H pylori infection is detected, preoperative therapy for eradication is advised.[23] The ASGE guidelines also state that patients without symptoms and who are not undergoing an endoscopy, if found positive for noninvasive H pylori, should be recommended for treatment.[8]

Liver and gall bladder

Liver histology in obese patients typically reveals significant abnormalities, including nonalcoholic fatty liver disease. Gastric bypass for obesity is associated with a dramatic improvement or normalization of liver histology in most patients. Therefore, liver disease should be assessed by the gastroenterologist preoperatively, usually with a combination of blood testing and imaging studies, such as ultrasonography. If cirrhosis is suspected, liver biopsy may be confirmatory. In one study, 73% of patients with confirmed histologic abnormalities of the liver before bariatric surgery had the changes normalize, and another 13% of patients had their abnormalities improve.[24]

Obesity is also associated with an increased prevalence of gallstones. Preoperative ultrasonography, as part of the evaluation of the GI tract before bariatric surgery, allows for detection of gallstones. If stones are present, the surgeon may consider a cholecystectomy at the same time as the bariatric procedure.[25,26]

SUMMARY

Preoperative evaluation of the GI tract before bariatric surgery yields important information that can lead to changes in planned treatments. Assessment may include upper endoscopy, which is indicated for many patients, testing for H pylori, and evaluation for preexisting liver and gall bladder disorders.

REFERENCES

1. Hedley AA, Ogden CL, Johnson CL, et al. Prevalence of overweight and obesity among US children, adolescents, and adults, 1999–2002. JAMA 2004;291:2847–50.

2. Bauchowitz AU, Gonder-Frederick LA, Olbrisch ME, et al. Psychosocial evaluation of bariatric surgery candidates:a survey of present practices. Psychosom Med 2005;67:825–32.
3. Still CD, Benotti P, Wood GC, et al. Outcomes of preoperative weight loss in high-risk patients undergoing gastric bypass surgery. Arch Surg 2007;142:994–8.
4. Colles SL, Dixon JB, Marks P, et al. Preoperative weight loss with a very-low-energy diet: quantitation of changes in liver and abdominal fat by serial imaging. Am J Clin Nutr 2006;84:304–11.
5. Lewis MC, Phillips ML, Slavotinek JP, et al. Change in liver size and fat content after treatment with Optifast very low calorie diet. Obes Surg 2006;16:697–701.
6. Kuruba R, Koche LS, Murr MM. Preoperative assessment and perioperative care of patients undergoing bariatric surgery. Med Clin North Am 2007;91:339–51.
7. SAGES Guidelines Committee. SAGES guideline for clinical application of laparoscopic bariatric surgery. Surg Endosc 2008;22:2281–300.
8. ASGE Standards of Practice Committee, Anderson MA, Gan SI, et al. Role of endoscopy in the bariatric surgery patient. Gastrointest Endosc 2008;68:1–10.
9. Muñoz R, Ibáñez L, Salinas J, et al. Importance of routine preoperative upper GI endoscopy: why all patients should be evaluated? Obes Surg 2009;19: 427–31.
10. Sharaf RN, Weinshel EH, Bini EJ, et al. Endoscopy plays an important preoperative role in bariatric surgery. Obes Surg 2004;14:1367–72.
11. Sevá-Pereira G, Trombeta VL. Early gastric cancer found at preoperative assessment for bariatric surgery. Obes Surg 2006;16:1109–11.
12. Korenkov M, Sauerland S, Shah S, et al. Is routine preoperative upper endoscopy in gastric banding patients really necessary? Obes Surg 2006;16:45–7.
13. Zeni TM, Frantzides CT, Mahr C, et al. Value of preoperative upper endoscopy in patients undergoing laparoscopic gastric bypass. Obes Surg 2006;16:142–6.
14. Verset D, Houben JJ, Gay F, et al. The place of upper gastrointestinal tract endoscopy before and after vertical banded gastroplasty for morbid obesity. Dig Dis Sci 1997;42:2333–7.
15. Hampel H, Abraham NS, El-Serag HB. Meta-analysis: obesity and the risk for gastroesophageal reflux disease and its complications. Ann Intern Med 2005; 143:199–211.
16. Schirmer B, Erenoglu C, Miller A. Flexible endoscopy in the management of patients undergoing Roux-en-Y gastric bypass. Obes Surg 2002;12:634–8.
17. Sauerland S, Angrisani L, Belachew M, et al. European Association for Endoscopic Surgery. Obesity surgery: evidence-based guidelines of the European Association for Endoscopic Surgery (EAES). Surg Endosc 2005;19:200–21.
18. Frigg A, Peterli R, Zynamon A, et al. Radiologic and endoscopic evaluation for laparoscopic adjustable gastric banding: preoperative and follow-up. Obes Surg 2001;11:594–9.
19. Fornari F, Gurski RR, Navarini D, et al. Clinical utility of endoscopy and barium swallow x-ray in the diagnosis of sliding hiatal hernia in morbidly obese patients: a study before and after gastric bypass. Obes Surg 2009. [Epub ahead of print].
20. Dhariwal A, Plevris JN, Lo NT, et al. Age, anemia, and obesity-associated oxygen desaturation during upper gastrointestinal endoscopy. Gastrointest Endosc 1992;38:684–8.
21. Madan AK, Tichansky DS, Isom J, et al. Monitored anesthesia care with propofol versus surgeon-monitored sedation with benzodiazepines and narcotics for preoperative endoscopy in the morbidly obese. Obes Surg 2008;18:545–8.

22. Azagury D, Dumonceau JM, Morel P, et al. Preoperative work-up in asymptomatic patients undergoing Roux-en-Y gastric bypass: is endoscopy mandatory? Obes Surg 2006;16:1304–11.
23. Csendes A, Burgos AM, Smok G, et al. Endoscopic and histologic findings of the foregut in 426 patients with morbid obesity. Obes Surg 2007;17:28–34.
24. Csendes A, Smok G, Burgos AM. Histological findings in the liver before and after gastric bypass. Obes Surg 2006;16:607–11.
25. Collazo-Clavell ML, Clark MM, et al. Assessment and preparation of patients for bariatric surgery. Mayo Clin Proc 2006;81:S11–7.
26. Escalona A, Boza C, Muñoz R, et al. Routine preoperative ultrasonography and selective cholecystectomy in laparoscopic Roux-en-Y gastric bypass. Why not? Obes Surg 2008;18:47–51.

Endoscopy in the Obese Patient

Mitchal A. Schreiner, MD, MPH, M. Brian Fennerty, MD*

KEYWORDS

• Endoscopy • Obese • Bariatric surgery • Gastrointestinal

Obese patients present many unique challenges to the endoscopist. Special consideration should be given to these patients, and endoscopists need to be aware of the additional challenges that may be present while performing endoscopic procedures on obese patients. This article reviews the special risks that obese patients face while undergoing endoscopy, endoscopic management of patients postbariatric surgery, and future role of endoscopy in the management of obese patients.

ENDOSCOPY IN OBESE PATIENTS: UNIQUE CHALLENGES
Upper Endoscopy in Obese Patients

As with all patients, it is important to ensure that an appropriate indication exists before performing endoscopy in obese patients. Obese patients are more likely than normal controls to have upper gastrointestinal (GI) symptoms, and hiatal hernias and gastritis are more likely identified by upper endoscopy.[1] It has also been shown that an elevated body mass index (BMI) is associated with an increased risk of adenocarcinoma of the esophagus and possibly gastric cardia.[2] In addition to increased risk for GI symptoms, obese patients also have an increased risk for underlying GI pathology. Therefore, there may be a lower threshold for performing endoscopy in obese patients despite the increased risk of the procedure related to their obesity.

Upper endoscopy is commonly recommended before performing bariatric surgery.[3,4] This is partly because of the fact that there is an increased prevalence of upper GI pathology in obese patients and that, depending on the bariatric surgery performed, the postsurgical anatomy may make future visualization of portions of the upper GI tract difficult, if not impossible. Furthermore, the endoscopic findings such as a large hiatal hernia, erosive esophagitis, or ulcer may alter the specific type of

Funding support: None.
Disclosures: None.
Division of Gastroenterology, Oregon Health and Science University, Mail Code L461, 3181 SW Sam Jackson Park Road, Portland, OR 97239, USA
* Corresponding author.
E-mail address: fennerty@ohsu.edu (M.B. Fennerty).

Gastroenterol Clin N Am 39 (2010) 87–97
doi:10.1016/j.gtc.2009.12.009
0889-8553/10/$ – see front matter © 2010 Elsevier Inc. All rights reserved.

gastro.theclinics.com

bariatric surgical procedure performed. As an example of the increase in associated pathology in obese patients, 1 study demonstrated that 42% of the subjects who underwent upper endoscopy before performing bariatric surgery required preoperative therapy for the pathology identified on their preoperative upper endoscopy.[5] However, this finding is not consistently found in the literature because another study demonstrated that routine upper endoscopy on subjects before bariatric surgery resulted in a change in the planned operative procedure in only 4.9% of cases.[6]

The American Society of Gastrointestinal Endoscopy has recently published guidelines regarding the use of endoscopy in patients before undergoing bariatric surgery. The recommendations in those guidelines are tailored to the bariatric procedure that is to be performed. They recommend the following:

(1) All patients with upper GI symptoms who are to undergo bariatric surgery should undergo a preoperative upper endoscopy.
(2) Upper endoscopy should be considered in all subjects who are to undergo Roux-en-Y gastric bypass (RYGB), regardless of the presence of symptoms.
(3) Preoperative upper endoscopy should be considered in asymptomatic patients before performing gastric banding to exclude large hiatal hernias because this may alter the surgical approach.[3]

The authors concur with these recommendations and emphasize that if routine screening upper endoscopy is not performed before bariatric surgery, the endoscopist will have a low threshold for performing upper endoscopy for symptom evaluation in prebariatric surgery patients.

Colonoscopy in Obese Patients

A case-control study has demonstrated a hazard ratio of 3.72 for the development of colon cancer in subjects with a BMI of more than 28,[7] and a prospective study revealed the rate ratio for colon cancer mortality in men with a BMI of more than 32.5 to be 1.9 and for women with a BMI of more than 32.5 to be 1.26.[8] Despite this increased risk of colon cancer prevalence and mortality in obese subjects, performing colonoscopy on patients with a high BMI can be challenging. It has been shown that obese patients are more likely to have an inadequate bowel preparation,[9] and the use of a more aggressive bowel preparation in obese subjects has been suggested. There has been a speculation that cecal intubation may be more difficult in obese patients (eg, difficulty in achieving adequate external pressure, repositioning of the patient); however, this does not appear to be the case because recent studies have actually shown cecal intubation to be more difficult in subjects with a lower BMI.[10] The authors have, however, found that the use of the longer enteroscope may help attain cecal intubation when there is difficulty intubating the cecum, which occurs as a result of looping or other factors during colonoscopy in obese patients. In addition, placing the obese patient in a prone position may improve cecal intubation time and reduce patient discomfort.[11]

Sedation Issues in Obese Patients

When an endoscopic procedure is indicated in an obese patient, there are several additional considerations that should be taken into account. One additional assessment of airway risk, although well accepted for anesthesia evaluation but not universally used in endoscopy, is the Mallampati score.[12] This score was originally devised to stratify risk related to endotracheal intubation, but it is also correlated with the risk of sleep apnea. The obese patient at risk for sleep apnea may also present an additional airway risk during endoscopy. Thus, the authors suggest that the endoscopist be aware of the possible utility of this scoring system in assessing the obese patient's risk for endoscopic sedation. It is also likely that the positioning of the patient further affects airway compromise in the obese patient more than it does in the nonobese. As such, performing the procedure with the patient in supine position may present greater airway risk in obese than in nonobese subjects.

It is also well established that obese patients are at an increased risk for sleep apnea,[13] and patients with sleep apnea are at an increased risk for developing cardio-vascular complications related to the use of sedation.[14] The authors completed a study of 397 subjects who underwent average-risk endoscopy at their institution and found that 35% had a BMI of more than 30, and 82% of those subjects were identified, by means of a validated sleep apnea questionnaire, as having high risk for sleep apnea. The study further revealed that subjects who were identified as having high risk for sleep apnea were more likely to have oxygen desaturation and hypercapnic episodes when undergoing sedation for standard, low-risk endoscopy. Based on these obser-vations, it was concluded that when a patient presents for endoscopy and sleep apnea is either suspected or confirmed, the endoscopist should use additional caution with the delivering and monitoring of sedation for endoscopy. Capnography may prove to be a helpful tool for monitoring these higher risk patients.

ENDOSCOPY IN OBESE PATIENTS: THE POSTBARIATRIC SURGERY PATIENT
Postbariatric Surgery Symptoms: When to Do Endoscopy?

Currently, the most common bariatric surgical procedures performed are the RYGB (**Fig. 1**) and laparoscopic adjustable gastric banding (LAGB) (**Fig. 2**). Other less commonly used procedures exist, such as vertical banded gastroplasty (VBG) (**Fig. 3**), sleeve gastrectomy (**Fig. 4**), and biliopancreatic diversion (**Fig. 5**). The varia-tion and extent of bariatric surgical procedures as well as marked differences in

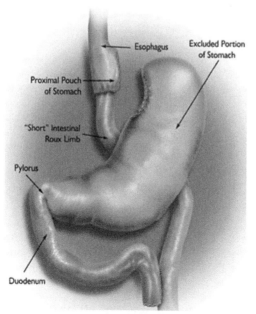

Fig. 1. Roux-en-Y gastric bypass. (*Courtesy of* Ethicon Endo-Surgery, Inc; with permission.)

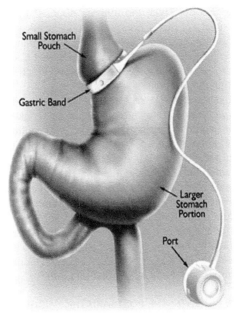

Fig. 2. Laparoscopic adjustable gastric band. (*Courtesy of* Ethicon Endo-Surgery, Inc; with permission.)

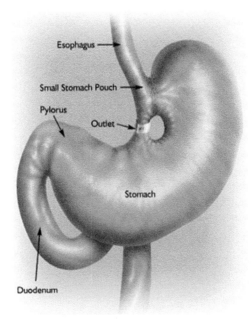

Fig. 3. Vertical banded gastroplasty. (*Courtesy of* Ethicon Endo-Surgery, Inc; with permission.)

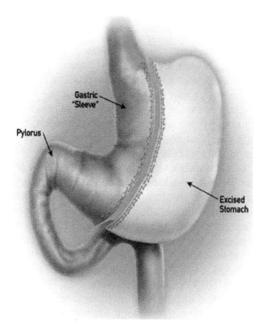

Fig. 4. Sleeve gastrectomy. (*Courtesy of* Ethicon Endo-Surgery, Inc; with permission.)

anatomy and complications associated with the various procedures mandate that endoscopists familiarize themselves with the surgical anatomy and complications before performing the procedure. Often it is helpful to speak directly with the surgeon who performed the procedure to clarify exactly what was done and the anatomic result

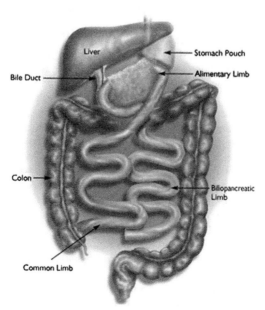

Fig. 5. Biliopancreatic diversion. (*Courtesy of* Ethicon Endo-Surgery, Inc; with permission.)

of the surgical procedure. If contact cannot be made, a detailed review of available surgical reports is warranted.

Upper GI symptoms are frequently seen in postbariatric surgery patients. The most common symptoms encountered are heartburn, regurgitation, dysphagia, nausea, vomiting, abdominal pain, persistent weight loss, and failure to lose weight or a plateau in weight loss that is less than expected.[5,15,16] The incidence of new reflux symptoms after bariatric surgery has not been well studied, and although there are some who believe that lap band surgery can worsen preoperative reflux, the preponderance of the literature suggests that gastroesophageal reflux disease symptoms are likely to improve after a bariatric surgical procedure is performed.[17-20]

Nausea, vomiting, or continued weight loss is often because of dietary noncompliance, such as rapid or large-volume food ingestion or inadequate chewing of ingested food, or the development of an anastomotic stricture. An early plateau in weight loss may also be because of dietary indiscretion or the development of anastomotic excessive dilation. Upper endoscopy should be considered (1) if upper GI symptoms are severe or persistent despite the patient eating an appropriate postsurgical diet, (2) if the patient begins to not tolerate a diet that had previously been tolerated at one point in the postoperative period, or (3) if weight loss is less than anticipated.

A prospective study of 1079 subjects who underwent RYGB revealed that significant pathology was identified in 68.4% of symptomatic patients referred for upper endoscopy.[15] The most common pathology identified was anastomotic stricture (52.6%), followed by marginal ulcer (15.8%), unraveled nonabsorbable sutures leading to functional obstruction (4%), and gastrogastric fistula (2.6%). Abnormal findings were seen in 85% of patients with dysphagia, 65% with nausea and/or vomiting, and 42% with abdominal pain. This study also noted that post-RYGB patients with an abnormal upper endoscopy had symptom onset at a mean of 110.7 days postprocedure compared with 347.5 days for patients with a normal upper endoscopy. In cases where a leak or fistula is suspected, one should start by getting an upper GI series, and if an abscess or seroma is suspected, a computed tomographic (CT) scan should be obtained before proceeding with endoscopy.

Management of Postbariatric Surgery Complications: Stenosis

The most common site of stenosis after bariatric surgery occurs at the gastrojejunal anastomosis after RYGB; however, other areas of stenosis have been described, including at the gastric band, area of passage through the mesocolon, jejunojejunal anastomosis, and at the site of adhesions. Studies have suggested that gastrojejunal anastomotic strictures occur in 5.1% to 6.8% of cases after RYGB,[21-23] and most occur within the first year after surgery. Endoscopic management of anastomotic strictures can be accomplished with through-the-scope balloon dilation or with Savary-Gilliard dilators (Cook Medical, Bloomington, IN, USA). An approach for the management of post-Roux-en-Y strictures has been proposed that takes into account the severity of the initial stenosis. This approach recommends (1) mild stenosis (able to pass 10.5-mm endoscope) be dilated to 16 to 18 mm with pneumatic dilation, (2) moderate stenosis (able to pass 8.5 mm endoscope) be managed with an initial pneumatic dilation up to 15 mm, followed 2 weeks later by dilation with Savary-Gilliard dilators up to 15 to 18 mm, and (3) severe stenosis (able to be traversed only with a wire guide) be dilated initially with a 6-mm balloon over a guidewire, with a maximum initial dilation not to exceed 10 mm, and subsequent dilations up to 15 mm with a Savary-Gilliard dilator depending on the success of previous dilations.[22]

There is some concern that dilation of strictures at the anastomosis can result in weight gain because of loss of the restrictive effect of the anastomosis; however, it has been shown that dilation of more than 15 mm does not appear to result in weight gain and most patients can have anastomotic narrowing managed with as few as 1 to 2 dilations.[21] When standard dilation is ineffective, additional strategies include cutting and removing exposed suture when present, injection of the anastomosis with saline or steroids postdilation, or even use of needle knife to disrupt scar tissue at the anastomosis site.

Management of Postbariatric Surgery Complications: Marginal Ulceration

Marginal or stomal ulceration occurs at the gastrojejunal anastomosis site, most frequently on the intestinal side of the anastomosis. Several predisposing factors have been proposed, including ischemia, use of nonsteroidal antiinflammatory drugs, staple line disruption, suture or staple erosion, gastrogastric fistula, and presence of *Helicobacter pylori*. Presence of *H pylori* preoperatively, even when adequately treated before surgery, increases the risk for marginal ulceration.[24] Because of the association of *H pylori* and postoperative ulcers, the American Society of Gastrointestinal Endoscopy has recommended that asymptomatic subjects who do not undergo preoperative endoscopy should undergo noninvasive *H pylori* testing, and if positive, they should be treated.[3] When a marginal ulceration is present, the endoscopist should give careful attention to inspecting the gastric pouch, as presence of a gastrogastric fistula can result in increased acid exposure to the pouch and the jejunum. This, along with the absence of the usual bicarbonate buffer in the proximal duodenum as a result of the patient's prior surgical procedure, may be a risk factor for ulcer formation. The role of endoscopy in dealing with marginal ulcers is typically for diagnosis; however, in cases where eroded suture material is present at the anastomosis, the suture material may be cut with endoscopic scissors and removed. Medical therapy for marginal ulcers consists of proton pump inhibitor therapy and sucralfate therapy, treatment of *H pylori* if found on biopsy, and avoidance of ulcerogenic medications. If the ulceration is particularly large or not responding to medical therapy, surgical revision may be required.

Management of Postbariatric Surgery Complications: Band Migration/Erosion and Slippage

The most common weight-loss surgical procedures that use a band that are encountered by endoscopists are the VBG and the LAGB. Gastric band erosion occurs in 1.6% to 3% of cases.[25,26] Gastric band erosion is best diagnosed endoscopically. If an eroded band is encountered, as long as it is encapsulated, it can be cut with endoscopic scissors and removed. If there is doubt about encapsulation, it can be confirmed with a CT scan. It should be noted that endoscopic removal of an eroded band cannot be performed with adjustable gastric bands because there is tubing present that connects the band to a subcutaneous port used for band adjustment. Removal of adjustable gastric bands thus requires surgical intervention. Gastric band slippage is another potential complication and is best diagnosed with an upper GI series. Endoscopically, gastric band slippage manifests as an enlarged pouch size and, in severe cases, may lead to ulceration or even gastric necrosis, a potentially life-threatening condition.

Management of Postbariatric Surgery Complications: Anastomotic Leaks and Fistulas

Studies have reported that anastomotic leaks after RYGB occur in 0% to 5.6% of cases[27,28] and are associated with high morbidity and mortality in the postsurgical patient. Anastomotic leaks generally present with abdominal pain, nausea, vomiting, fever, and tachycardia and are best diagnosed with an upper GI series. Intraoperative endoscopy has been proposed as a way to identify leaks intraoperatively so that they may be surgically repaired before completing the surgical procedure. In one study, intraoperative endoscopy was performed on 825 consecutive patients undergoing laparoscopic bariatric procedures and 3.5% of the patients were found to have leaks that were then surgically corrected.[29] In cases where chronic leaks or fistulas develop, surgical revision is often required. However, less-invasive endoscopic approaches have been described. Partially covered self-expanding metal stents, polyflex stents, argon plasma coagulation, endoclips, distal gastrojejunal stenosis dilation, and fibrin glue have all been used in the treatment of chronic leaks and fistulas.[30,31]

Management of Postbariatric Surgery Complications: Loss of Effect of Surgery

Failure to lose weight or regaining previously lost weight after bariatric surgery may be the result of ingestion of high-calorie liquids or soft foods, gastric pouch dilation, large patulous gastrojejunal anastomosis, and gastrogastric fistula formation. Endoscopic therapies to reduce the size of a patulous gastrojejunal anastomosis have been described. One approach is to perform 4-quadrant injections of sodium morrhuate to induce scarring at the anastomosis.[32] Another approach involves endoscopic placement and tightening of sutures at the rim of the gastrojejunal anastomosis leading to tissue placations, thus reducing the diameter of the anastomosis and potentially the size of the gastric pouch.[33] Strategies for endoscopic management of gastrogastric fistulas have already been described earlier.

ENDOSCOPY IN OBESE PATIENTS: FUTURE ROLE OF ENDOSCOPY
Endoscopic Bariatric Procedures

At present there is significant interest in developing safe and effective endoscopic bariatric procedures; however, no such approaches have yet been perfected. Human studies have been performed investigating the use of an intragastric balloon, and transoral gastroplasty. A short-term randomized controlled study found that the use of an intragastric balloon in morbidly obese patients resulted in significant weight loss when the intragastric balloon was in place for a 3-month period.[34] Another study looking at the use of an intragastric balloon found that use for more than a 1-year time period resulted in substantial weight loss, which was maintained by most patients during the following year after the intragastric balloon was removed.[35]

Endoscopic gastroplasty has been performed with the use of endoscopic stapling and endoscopic suturing. In a study using transoral endoscopically guided staplers, a restrictive gastric pouch was created along the lesser curvature of the stomach in 11 patients. This resulted in a decrease in the average BMI from 41.6 to 33.1 for more than a 3-month period, with no major adverse events noted.[36] Another study used endoscopic suturing to perform endoluminal vertical gastroplasty in 64 patients. Follow-up after 1 year postprocedure revealed a decrease in the mean BMI from 39.9 to 30.6, and no serious adverse events occurred.[37]

SUMMARY

- Obese patients are at an increased risk for upper and lower GI pathology, and endoscopists should have a decreased threshold for performing endoscopic procedures on obese patients.
- Because of the increased risk of sleep apnea in obese patients, extra caution should be used while administering sedation for endoscopic procedures in obese patients.

- Before bariatric surgery, in centers where routine prebariatric surgery upper endoscopy is not performed, all patients with upper GI symptoms should receive a preoperative upper endoscopy.
- Because the postsurgical anatomy makes endoscopic evaluation difficult, preoperative endoscopy should be considered in patients who are to undergo RYGB, regardless of the presence or absence of symptoms.
- Consider performing preoperative endoscopy on patients before proceeding with gastric banding, as large hiatal hernias may require an alteration in the surgical approach.
- Asymptomatic subjects who do not undergo preoperative endoscopy should undergo noninvasive *H pylori* testing, and if positive, they should be treated.
- Endoscopy plays a key role in the diagnosis and treatment of the complications arising from bariatric surgery.
- Upper endoscopy should be performed in all postbariatric surgery patients who have persistent or severe symptoms despite following a recommended postsurgical diet, and if a leak is suspected, a contrast radiographic study should be performed first.
- The most common complications of bariatric surgery include gastrojejunal anastomotic stricture, marginal ulceration, band migration and slippage, anastomotic leak and fistula formation, and loss of surgical effect.
- Studies suggest that endoscopic bariatric procedures may be safe and effective and may become commonplace in the future.

REFERENCES

1. Dutta SK, Arora M, Kireet A, et al. Upper gastrointestinal symptoms and associated disorders in morbidly obese patients: a prospective study. Dig Dis Sci 2009; 54:1243–6.
2. Kubo A, Corley D. Body mass index and adenocarcinomas of the esophagus or gastric cardia: a systematic review and meta-analysis. Cancer Epidemiol Biomarkers Prev 2006;15:872–8.
3. Anderson MA, Gan SI, Fanelli RD, et al. Role of endoscopy in the bariatric surgery patient. Gastrointest Endosc 2008;68:1–10.
4. Sauerland S, Angrisani L, Belachew M, et al. European association for endoscopic surgery. Obesity surgery: evidence-based guidelines of the European Association for Endoscopic Surgery (EAES). Surg Endosc 2005;19:200–21.
5. Verset D, Houben JJ, Gay F, et al. The place of upper gastrointestinal tract endoscopy before and after vertical banded gastroplasty for morbid obesity. Dig Dis Sci 1997;42:2333–7.
6. Schirmer B, Erenoglu C, Miller A. Flexible endoscopy in the management of patients undergoing Roux-en-Y gastric bypass. Obes Surg 2002;12:634–8.
7. Boutron-Ruault MC, Senesse P, Meance S, et al. Energy intake, body mass index, physical activity, and the colorectal adenoma-carcinoma sequence. Nutr Cancer 2001;39:50–7.
8. Murphy TK, Calle EE, Rodriguez C, et al. Body mass index and colon cancer mortality in a large prospective study. Am J Epidemiol 2000;152:847–54.
9. Borg BB, Gupta NK, Zukerman GR, et al. Impact of obesity on bowel preparation for colonoscopy. Clin Gastroenterol Hepatol 2009;7:670–5.
10. Krishnan P, Demsey R, Nawras A. Does size really matter? A prospective study to evaluate body habitus and difficulty level of colonoscopy. Gastrointest Endosc 2008;67:AB245.

11. Desormeaux M, Scicluna M, Friedland S. Colonoscopy in obese patients: a growing problem. Gastrointest Endosc 2008;67:AB89.
12. Nuckton TJ, Glidden DV, Browner WS, et al. Physical examination: Mallampati score as an independent predictor of obstructive sleep apnea. Sleep 2006;29: 903–8.
13. Tishler PV, Larkin EK, Schluchter MD, et al. Incidence of sleep-disordered breathing in an urban adult population. JAMA 2003;289:2230–7.
14. Chung SA, Yuan H, Chung F. A systemic review of obstructive sleep apnea and Its implications for anesthesiologists. Anesth Analg 2008;107:1543–63.
15. Lee JK, Van Dam J, Morton JM, et al. Endoscopy is accurate, safe, and effective in the assessment and management of complications following gastric bypass surgery. Am J Gastroenterol 2009;104:575–82.
16. DeMaria EJ, Sugerman HJ, Meador JG, et al. High failure rate after laparoscopic adjustable silicone gastric banding for treatment of morbid obesity. Ann Surg 2001;233:809–18.
17. Smith SC, Edwards CB, Goodman GN. Symptomatic and clinical improvement in morbidly obese patients with gastroesophageal reflux disease following Roux-en-Y gastric bypass. Obes Surg 1997;7:479–84.
18. Spivak H, Hewitt MF, Onn A, et al. Weight loss and improvement of obesity-related illness in 500 U.S. patients following laparoscopic adjustable gastric banding procedure. Am J Surg 2005;189:27–32.
19. Clements RH, Gonzalez QH, Foster A, et al. Gastrointestinal symptoms are more intense in morbidly obese patients and are improved with laparoscopic Roux-en-Y gastric bypass. Obes Surg 2003;13:610–4.
20. Tolonen P, Victorzon M, Niemi R, et al. Does gastric banding for morbid obesity reduce or increase gastroesophageal reflux? Obes Surg 2006;16:1469–74.
21. Peifer KJ, Shields AJ, Azar R, et al. Successful endoscopic management of gastrojejunal anastomotic strictures after Roux-en-Y gastric bypass. Gastrointest Endosc 2007;66:248–52.
22. Goitein D, Papasavas PK, Gagne D, et al. Gastrojejunal strictures following laparoscopic Roux-en-Y gastric bypass for morbid obesity. Surg Endosc 2005;19: 628–32.
23. Go MR, Muscarella P, Needleman BJ, et al. Endoscopic management of stomal stenosis after Roux-en-Y gastric bypass. Surg Endosc 2004;18:56–9.
24. Rasmussen JJ, Fuller W, Ali MR. Marginal ulceration after laparoscopic gastric bypass: an analysis of predisposing factors in 260 patients. Surg Endosc 2007;21:190–4.
25. Nocca D, Frering V, Gallix B, et al. Migration of adjustable gastric banding from a cohort study of 4236 patients. Surg Endosc 2005;19:947–50.
26. Stroh C, Hohmann U, Will U, et al. Experiences of two centers of bariatric surgery in the treatment of intragastrale band migration after gastric banding – the importance of the German multicenter observational study for quality assurance in obesity surgery 2005 and 2006. Int J Colorectal Dis 2008;23:901–8.
27. Higda KD, Boone KB, Ho T. Complications of the laparoscopic Roux-en-Y gastric bypass: 1040 patients – What have we learned? Obes Surg 2000;10: 509–13.
28. Fernandez AZ, DeMaria EJ, Tichansky DS. Experience with over 3000 open and laparoscopic bariatric procedures: multivariate analysis of factors related to leak and resultant mortality. Surg Endosc 2004;18:193–7.
29. Champion JK, Hunt T, DeLisle N. Role of routine intraoperative endoscopy in laparoscopic bariatric surgery. Surg Endosc 2002;16:1663–5.

30. Eisendrath P, Cremer M, Himpens J, et al. Endotherapy including temporary stenting of fistulas of the upper gastrointestinal tract after laparoscopic bariatric surgery. Endoscopy 2007;39:625–30.
31. Merrifield BF, Lautz D, Thompson CC. Endoscopic repair of gastric leaks after Roux-en-Y gastric bypass: a less invasive approach. Gastrointest Endosc 2006;63:710–4.
32. Catalano MF, Rudic G, Anderson AJ, et al. Weight gain following bariatric surgery as a result of a large gastric stoma: endotherapy with sodium morrhuate may prevent the need for surgical revision. Gastrointest Endosc 2007;66:240–5.
33. Thompson CC, Slattery J, Bundga ME, et al. Peroral endoscopic reduction of dilated gastrojejunal anastomosis after Roux-en-Y gastric bypass: a possible new option for patients with weight regain. Surg Endosc 2006;20:1744–8.
34. Genco A, Cipriano M, Bacci V, et al. BioEnterics Intragastric Balloon (BIB): a short term, double-blind, randomised, controlled, crossover study on weight reduction in morbidly obese patients. Int J Obes 2006;30:129–33.
35. Mathus-Vliegen EM, Tytgat GN. Intragastric balloon for treatment-resistant obesity: safety, tolerance, and efficacy of 1-year balloon treatment followed by a 1-year balloon-free follow-up. Gastrointest Endosc 2005;61:19–27.
36. Moreno C, Closset J, Dugardeyn S, et al. Transoral gastroplasty is safe, feasible, and induces significant weight loss in morbidly obese patients: results of the second human pilot study. Endoscopy 2008;40:406–13.
37. Fogel R, De Fogel J, Bonilla Y, et al. Clinical experience of transoral suturing for an endoluminal vertical gastroplasty: 1-year follow up in 64 patients. Gastrointest Endosc 2008;68:51–8.

Endoscopic Retrograde Cholangiopancreatography in Patients with Roux-en-Y Anatomy

Tercio L. Lopes, MD, MSPH[a],*, C. Mel Wilcox, MD, MSPH[b]

KEYWORDS

• Bariatric • Duodenoscope • Cannulation • Roux-en-Y anatomy

Bariatric surgery has been increasingly performed in response to the obesity pandemic. During the last decade, Roux-en-Y gastric bypass (RYGB) has become the preferred surgical approach, presently accounting for more than two-thirds of about 150,000 such procedures performed annually in the United States.[1] In addition, Roux-en-Y reconstruction is also commonly performed after pylorus-preserving pancreaticoduodenectomy and other biliary tract surgeries. Consequently, endoscopists are now often faced with the need to carry out endoscopic examinations and therapeutic interventions in patients with Roux-en-Y anatomy.

Roux-en-Y anatomy poses a serious challenge to endoscopists when access to the biliary tree or the pancreas is required. In patients with this anatomy, an endoscope advanced through the anatomic route needs first to reach the jejunojejunostomy, and subsequently make its way up the biliopancreatic limb until the papilla or the bilioenteric (BE)/pancreatoenteric (PE) anastomosis is reached. The distance from the jejunojejunostomy to the papilla varies greatly depending on the indication for the Roux-en-Y reconstruction. It is typically the maximum after bariatric surgery, frequently exceeding 80 to 100 cm. The distance of the bowel to be traversed certainly affects the success rate of the endoscopic retrograde cholangiopancreatography (ERCP), which is performed by advancing an endoscope through the anatomic route.

This article discusses the different options available for endoscopists who are faced with the need to perform ERCP in patients post–Roux-en-Y reconstruction, with special emphasis on those patients post-RYGB.

[a] Division of Gastroenterology and Hepatology, Mayo Clinic College of Medicine, 200 First Street SW, Rochester, MN 55905, USA
[b] Division of Gastroenterology and Hepatology, University of Alabama at Birmingham, Birmingham, 703 19th Street South, ZRB 633 Birmingham, AL 35294, USA
* Corresponding author.
E-mail address: Lopes.Tercio@mayo.edu

Gastroenterol Clin N Am 39 (2010) 99–107
doi:10.1016/j.gtc.2009.12.008
0889-8553/10/$ – see front matter © 2010 Elsevier Inc. All rights reserved.

gastro.theclinics.com

ADVANCEMENT OF DUODENOSCOPES THROUGH THE ANATOMIC ROUTE

The side-viewing duodenoscope is the ideal instrument to perform ERCP, particularly for the cannulation of a native papilla. Nevertheless, advancement of the duodenoscope through the anatomic route is frequently unsuccessful in patients with Roux-en-Y anatomy. For example, Hintze and colleagues[2] reported a 33% success rate for reaching the papilla with a duodenoscope in patients with short-limb Roux-en-Y anatomy (none post-RYGB). Wright and colleagues[3] reported the largest series of patients with Roux-en-Y anatomy and intact papilla who underwent ERCP after advancement of colonoscopes or duodenoscopes through the per os anatomic route. Their approach consisted of an initial exploration of the afferent limb with a forward-viewing colonoscope and an attempted cannulation. If cannulation was not achieved via the colonoscope, a guidewire was placed into the excluded stomach or duodenum to guide the advancement of a duodenoscope, which was inserted over the guidewire under fluoroscopic guidance. On some occasions, an over-the-wire balloon dilator was used to anchor the guidewire to the afferent limb, facilitating the advancement of the duodenoscope. The investigators used techniques similar to those used during colonoscopy to facilitate advancement of the duodeno-scope, including alternating advancement and withdrawal with straightening of loops, turning the patient to the left lateral or supine position, and compression of the abdomen. Fifteen patients underwent attempted ERCP using these techniques (11 post-RYGB, 4 postgastric resection). ERCP was possible in 10 patients (67%), some of whom had repeated procedures. Use of the colonoscope was successful in 2 patients (13%), and use of the duodenoscope was successful in 8 patients (53%). Interventions performed included sphincter of Oddi manometry, biliary sphinc-terotomy, stone extraction, and placement of pancreatic and biliary stents. ERCP was not possible in 5 patients (33%), all of whom had undergone RYGB. All 5 patients in whom the initial attempt to reach the papilla failed underwent a second attempt (1 patient underwent a third attempt), all without success. In contrast, repeated attempts were always successful in those patients in whom the insertion of the endoscope was successful at the first attempt. The large number of failed procedures, even in very experienced hands, underscores the challenges of performing ERCP through the anatomic route in patients with Roux-en-Y anatomy.

ADVANCEMENT OF ENTEROSCOPES OR COLONOSCOPES THROUGH THE PER OS ANATOMIC ROUTE

The use of a pediatric colonoscope (without surgical assistance) to perform ERCP in patients with Roux-en-Y anatomy was first reported by Gostout and Bender[4] in 1989. Roux-en-Y anatomy was a consequence of gastrectomy for peptic ulcer disease in 2 patients and hepaticojejunostomy for biliary-cutaneous fistula in 1 patient. No patient had undergone bariatric surgery. Two patients had a history of BE anastomosis (hep-aticojejunostomy and choledochoduodenostomy), whereas 1 patient had a native papilla. ERCP was successfully performed in all patients, although percutaneous transhepatic cholangiography was initially necessary to guide cannulation in the patient who had a choledochoduodenostomy.

Elton and colleagues[5] reported their experience with 18 patients with Roux-en-Y anatomy who underwent 25 attempts of ERCP. Of those, 3 patients had undergone RYGB (length of the bypassed segment unknown). Successful insertion to the level of the papilla or PE/BE anastomosis was possible in 86% of patients with an entero-scope and in 82% with a pediatric colonoscope. Biliary cannulation was successful in 4 of 5 patients with native papilla, and pancreatic cannulation was successful in 50%

of the patients. In experienced hands, pediatric colonoscopes and enteroscopes can be successfully used to perform ERCP in patients with a short Roux limb and in those with BE/PE anastomosis. However, only selected reports are available describing cannulation of an intact papilla in patients post-RYGB.[5,6] To the authors' knowledge, there is no prospective analysis of the success rate of ERCP performed with a colonoscope or enteroscope in patients post-RYGB.

ERPC WITH DOUBLE- OR SINGLE-BALLOON ENTEROSCOPES

As double-balloon enteroscopy (DBE) and single-balloon enteroscopy (SBE) have become more widely available, an increasing number of reports have emerged describing their use for performing ERCP in patients with Roux-en-Y anatomy. Balloon-assisted enteroscopy offers the advantage of reducing loops of small bowel over the endoscope, facilitating progression through the anatomic route in patients post–Roux-en-Y reconstruction. In fact, centers with experience in DBE have reported a success rate greater than 90% for reaching the biliopancreatic limb in patients with Roux-en-Y anatomy and a combined 80% success rate for ERCP.[7–16] In a recent series of 13 patients, Neumann and colleagues[17] reported a success rate of 61% for reaching the biliopancreatic limb with SBE and 46% for performing ERCP.

Although the high success rates with DBE are encouraging, most of the experience with the technique involved patients with hepaticojejunostomy. Similar to enteroscopes and colonoscopes, forward-viewing DBE is not ideal for the cannulation of a native papilla. Furthermore, it is unclear if DBE performs as well in patients with longer Roux limbs (eg, post-RYGB). The lack of therapeutic instruments long enough for use with the DBE is also a major limitation.[9]

ERCP THROUGH GASTROSTOMY OR JEJUNOSTOMY TRACTS

In 1998, Baron and Vickers[18] reported the first case of surgical gastrostomy placement as a means of access for diagnostic and therapeutic ERCP in a patient post-RYGB experiencing recurrent pancreatitis. After a failed attempt at ERCP with an enteroscope (papilla could not be reached), the investigators obtained access to the excluded stomach via a surgical gastrostomy. Initially, open Stamm gastrostomy of the distal stomach was performed with the placement of a 24F Malecot tube. The gastrostomy tube was removed 2 weeks later, and a 7.9-mm diameter pediatric forward-viewing endoscope was inserted through the gastrostomy site into the distal stomach and the duodenum. Dilation was performed with Savary dilators over a wire to 38F. Immediately after dilatation, ERCP was performed with a diagnostic duodenoscope. Biliary and pancreatic cannulation as well as biliary and pancreatic manometry were performed. Biliary and pancreatic sphincterotomy were performed to treat sphincter of Oddi dysfunction (SOD).

After that initial report, other investigators have described their experience with the technique in patients with Roux-en-Y anatomy.[19–22] Matlock and colleagues[19] have reported 14 patients who underwent ERCP through gastrostomy tracts. In 13 patients, ERCP was performed intraoperatively with a sterile duodenoscope, immediately after surgical placement of the gastrostomy; Of 14 gastrostomies, 10 were placed laparoscopically. Success rates for attempted ERCP was 100% for biliary cannulation (25/25), biliary manometry (10/10), biliary sphincterotomy (14/14), pancreatic duct cannulation (19/19), pancreatic sphincterotomy (15/15), a minor papilla cannulation and papillotomy (1).

Although gastrostomy offers reliable access with a side-viewing duodenoscope, this technique is more invasive than other purely endoscopic approaches and is associated with risks related to anesthesia and surgery. Feeding tubes left in place offer the option of access when the need for repeated procedures is anticipated. Nevertheless, the presence of feeding tubes may also raise issues related to body image and discomfort associated with activities of daily living.[23] For this reason, gastrostomy tubes should be removed after ERCP as soon as feasible. Unless ERCP is performed intraoperatively, it may be impractical to wait for the gastrostomy tract to mature (such as in a patient with cholangitis).

LAPAROSCOPIC-ASSISTED ERCP

Laparoscopic creation of a point of access to the gastric remnant or the small bowel allows for a duodenoscope to reach the papilla (or BE/PE anastomosis) when ERCP is indicated in patients with Roux-en-Y anatomy. Once such access to the excluded stomach or to the small bowel is established, the endoscopist inserts a previously sterilized duodenoscope through a 15-mm trocar and observes as it exits into the peritoneum. The surgeon and the endoscopist work collaboratively to guide the endoscope into the excluded stomach (or biliopancreatic limb) (**Figs. 1** and **2**). The endoscope is then advanced through the pylorus and positioned in the second duodenum, similar to a standard ERCP. Endoscopy technicians assist the endoscopist during the procedure, working independently from the operating room staff (**Figs. 3** and **4**). Although laparoscopic-assisted ERCP (LAERCP) is not yet widely performed, the reported experience with this technique is steadily growing. Reports of 20 patients who have undergone successful LAERCP are available in the literature (attempted in 21, technical success of 95%).[24–31] The failed procedure was because of stone impaction in the ampulla, which prevented cannulation.[27] Therapeutic interventions, such as biliary sphincterotomy (n = 20),[24–31] stone extraction (n = 7),[26,27,29–31] sphincter of Oddi manometry (n = 2),[9] and endoscopic closure of a gastrogastric fistula (n = 1), are typically performed after laparoscopic-assisted access.[31] No complications have been reported.

The authors have submitted their experience with 10 patients who underwent LAERCP at the University of Alabama at Birmingham.[32] Of these, 9 patients had undergone RYGB, whereas 1 had a history of partial gastrectomy with Roux-en-Y reconstruction. Indications for LAERCP were (1) choledocholithiasis (n = 4, 40%), (2) suspected biliary stricture (n = 3, 30%) and (3) suspected SOD type 1 (n = 3,

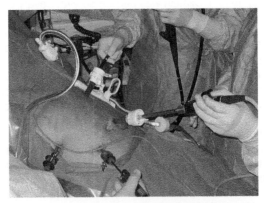

Fig. 1. Operation field during laparoscopic-assisted ERCP. The endoscope is introduced through a 15-mm laparoscopic trocar into the excluded stomach or the small bowel.

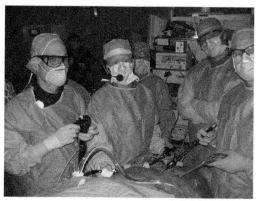

Fig. 2. The endoscopist and the surgical team work collaboratively to position the duodeno-scope and to carry out the procedure.

30%). Biliary cannulation was successfully performed in 9 of 10 patients (90%); pancreatic cannulation in 3 of 3 patients (100%). All patients underwent biliary sphinc-terotomy, but pancreatic sphincterotomy was not performed. Two patients underwent sphincter of Oddi manometry, and in 1 patient a 3F pancreatic stent was placed prophylactically (chosen because these almost invariably pass spontaneously). During the laparoscopic examination, internal hernias were diagnosed and treated in 4 patients. An additional patient was treated surgically for symptomatic adhesions. A patient with a previously placed percutaneous transhepatic cholangiography catheter still in place developed a tension pneumothorax during the procedure, as gas tracked along the catheter into the right pleural space. Fortunately, this was promptly recog-nized, and the patient immediately responded to the placement of a small-bore chest tube, allowing the procedure to be completed successfully.

Although LAERCP is reliably successful, the approach is associated with the inherent risks of anesthesia and surgery. Compared with the purely endoscopic approaches and gastrostomy access (particularly when tube is placed percutane-ously), LAERCP offers the benefits of laparoscopic examination of the abdominal cavity and of the ability to diagnose and treat internal hernias. This is an important

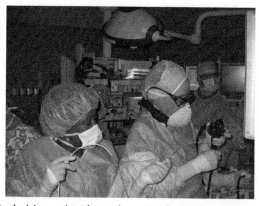

Fig. 3. Endoscopy technician assists the endoscopist during laparoscopic-assisted ERCP.

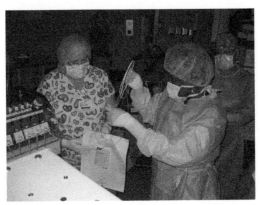

Fig. 4. Endoscopy technicians prepare for sphincter of Oddi manometry.

complication, in view of the high incidence of internal hernias (ranging from 0.2%–9%) in patients post-RYGB.[33,34] When the need for repeated access is anticipated, placement of a gastrostomy tube should be strongly considered.

CHOOSING THE BEST APPROACH

To determine the best technique to perform ERCP in a patient with Roux-en-Y anatomy, an endoscopist must

1. Understand the anatomy of the patient (long vs short Roux limb, native papilla vs BE/PE anastomosis).
2. Consider the indication for ERCP (likelihood of repeat procedures, need for manometry, need for needle-knife sphincterotomy, possibility of internal hernia).
3. Assess surgical risk.
4. Employ local expertise (DBE/SBE/Spirus, interventional radiologists, surgeons).

Table 1 summarizes the characteristics of the different approaches for ERCP in patients with Roux-en-Y anatomy. In patients with native papilla, techniques that rely on forward-viewing endoscopes are suboptimal. If a short roux limb is anticipated, advancement of a duodenoscope through the anatomic route can be attempted, although this approach is laborious and frequently unsuccessful. LAERCP and gastrostomy access are the authors' preferred approaches in patients fit for surgery, particularly in those with long Roux limbs (such as post-RYGB). If internal hernias are suspected, LAERCP has a distinct advantage; if repeated access is a possibility, gastrostomy tube access is ideal. In poor surgical candidates, percutaneously placed gastrostomy tubes or percutaneous interventions by a skilled radiologist may be the best option.

Forward-viewing endoscopes are often successful when ERCP is to be performed in a patient who has undergone BE/PE anastomosis. Although enteroscopes and colonoscopes can be used in patients with short Roux limbs,[4,5] according to the authors' experience, they are unlikely to be successful in patients with long Roux limbs. Similarly, SBE seems to have lower success rates in patients post-RYGB.[17] DBE, if available, is a reasonable approach for ERCP in patients with a long Roux limb, particularly in those with BE/PE anastomosis. When SBE/DBE is considered, the endoscopist must anticipate the need for therapeutic instruments, which are of limited availability for these endoscopes.

Table 1
Comparison of the different approaches for ERPC in patients with Roux-en-Y anatomy

Technique	Advantages	Disadvantages	Best Application
Duodenoscope through anatomic route	Side-viewing endoscope facilitates cannulation and therapy of native papillas Minimally invasive	Time consuming Often unsuccessful	Patients with native papilla and short Roux limb
Colonoscope/ enteroscope through anatomic route	Minimally invasive	Time consuming Often unsuccessful in long Roux limb	BE/PE anastomosis and short Roux limb
Single/double-balloon enteroscopes	Minimally invasive High success rates	Forward viewing Limited availability of instruments	BE/PE (short/long Roux limb)
ERCP through gastrostomy/ jejunostomy	Access with side-viewing duodenoscope Allows for repeat procedures	More invasive than purely endoscopic approaches	RYGB with native papilla, when internal hernias not likely or when repeat procedures anticipated
LAERCP	Access with side-viewing duodenoscope Laparoscopy can diagnose and treat internal hernias	More invasive than purely endoscopic approaches	RYGB, particularly when internal hernia is in the differential diagnosis
Interventional radiology	Less invasive than surgical approaches	Morbidity (pain, external drains) No access to pancreas	Patients with biliary pathology, unfit to undergo surgery

As the number of RYGB procedures continues to increase in the United States and worldwide, endoscopists will increasingly face the need to perform ERCP in patients with Roux-en-Y anatomy. Several techniques are available to assist endoscopists in conquering this challenging task. Nevertheless, no single approach will fit the needs of all patients. By understanding the surgical anatomy, carefully planning all steps of the procedure, assessing the patient's surgical risk, and making use of local expertise, endoscopists will greatly increase their chance of success and will certainly improve the quality of care delivered to their patients with surgically altered anatomy.

REFERENCES

1. Schauer P, Ikramuddin S. Laparoscopic surgery for morbid obesity. Surg Clin North Am 2001;81:1145–79.
2. Hintze RE, Adler A, Veltzke W, et al. Endoscopic access to the papilla of Vater for endoscopic retrograde cholangiopancreatolgraphy in patients with Billroth II or Roux-en-Y gastrojejunostomy. Endoscopy 1997;29:69–73.
3. Wright BE, Cass OW, Freeman ML. ERCP in patients with long-limb Roux-en-Y gastrojejunostomy and intact papilla. Gastrointest Endosc 2002;56:225–32.

4. Gostout CJ, Bender CE. Cholangiopancreatography, sphincterotomy, and common bile duct stone removal via Roux-en-Y limb enteroscopy. Gastroenterology 1988;95:156–63.
5. Elton E, Hanson BL, Qaseem T, et al. Diagnostic and therapeutic ERCP using an enteroscope and pediatric colonoscope in long-limb surgical bypass patients. Gasrtointest Endosc 1998;47:62–7.
6. Mosca S, Uomo G, Ceglia T, et al. Is it always true that ERCP cannot be carried out in patients with Roux-en-Y gastrojejunosotmy? [letter]. Endoscopy 1998;30:870.
7. Mönkemüller K, Fry LC, Bellutti M, et al. ERCP using single-balloon instead of double-balloon enteroscopy in patients with Roux-en-Y anastomosis. Endoscopy 2008;40:E19–20.
8. Chu YC, Yang CC, Yeh YH, et al. Double-balloon enteroscopy application in biliary tract disease-its therapeutic and diagnostic functions. Gastrointest Endosc 2008;68:585–91.
9. Koornstra JJ. Double balloon enteroscopy for endoscopic retrograde cholangio-pancreaticography after Roux-en-Y reconstruction: case series and review of the literature. Neth J Med 2008;66:275–9.
10. Aabakken L, Bretthauer M, Line PD. Double-balloon enteroscopy for endoscopic retrograde cholangiography in patients with a Roux-en-Y anastomosis. Endoscopy 2007;39:1068–71.
11. Haruta H, Yamamoto H, Mizuta K, et al. A case of successful enteroscopic balloon dilation for late anastomotic stricture of choledochojejunostomy after living donor liver transplantation. Liver Transpl 2005;11:1608–10.
12. Emmett DS, Mallat DB. Double-balloon ERCP in patients who have undergone Roux-en-Y surgery: a case series. Gastrointest Endosc 2007;66:1038–41.
13. Moreels TG, Roth B, Vandervliet EJ, et al. The use of the double-balloon enteroscope for endoscopic retrograde cholangiopancreatography and biliary stent placement after Roux-en-Y hepaticojejunostomy. Endoscopy 2007;39:E196–7.
14. Spahn TW, Grosse-Thie W, Spies P, et al. Treatment of choledocholithiasis following Roux-en-Y hepaticojejunostomy using double-balloon endoscopy. Digestion 2007;75:20–1.
15. Mönkemüller K, Bellutti M, Neumann H, et al. Therapeutic ERCP with the double-balloon enteroscope in patients with Roux-en-Y anastomosis. Gastrointest Endosc 2008;67:992–6.
16. Parlak E, Ciçek B, Dişibeyaz S, et al. Endoscopic retrograde cholangiography by double balloon enteroscopy in patients with Roux-en-Y hepaticojejunostomy. Surg Endosc 2009. [Epub ahead of print].
17. Neumann H, Fry LC, Meyer F, et al. Endoscopic retrograde cholangiopancreatography using the single balloon enteroscope technique in patients with Roux-en-Y anastomosis. Digestion 2009;80:52–7.
18. Baron TH, Vickers SM. Surgical gastrostomy placement as access for diagnostic and therapeutic ERCP. Gastrointest Endosc 1998;48:640–1.
19. Matlock J, Ikramuddin S, Lederer H, et al. Bypassing the bypass: ERCP via gastrostomy after bariatric surgery. Gastrointest Endosc 2005;61:AB98.
20. Martinez J, Guerrero L, Byers P, et al. Endoscopic retrograde cholangiopancreatography and gastroduodenoscopy after Roux-en-Y gastric bypass. Surg Endosc 2006;20:1548–50.
21. Baron TH, Chahal P, Ferreira LE. ERCP via mature feeding jejunostomy tube tract in a patient with Roux-en-Y anatomy. Gastrointest Endosc 2008;68:189–91.

22. Brotherton AM, Judd PA. Quality of life in adult enteral tube feeding patients. J Hum Nutr Diet 2007;20:513–22.
23. Bannerman E, Pendlebury J, Phillips F, et al. A cross-sectional and longitudinal study of health-related quality of life after percutaneous gastrostomy. Eur J Gastroenterol Hepatol 2000;12:1101–9.
24. Peters M, Papasavas PK, Caushaj PF, et al. Laparoscopic transgastric endoscopic retrograde cholangiopancreatography for benign common bile duct stricture after Roux-en-Y gastric bypass. Surg Endosc 2002;16:1106.
25. Pimentel RR, Mehran A, Szomstein S, et al. Laparoscopy-assisted transgastrostomy ERCP after bariatric surgery: case report of a novel approach. Gastrointest Endosc 2004;59:325–8.
26. Nguyen NT, Hinojosa MW, Slone J, et al. Laparoscopic transgastric access to the biliary tree after Roux-en-Y bypass. Obes Surg 2007;17:416–9.
27. Ceppa FA, Gagné DJ, Papasavas PK, et al. Laparoscopic transgastric endoscopy after Roux-en-Y gastric bypass. Surg Obes Relat Dis 2007;3:21–4.
28. Nakao FS, Mendes CJ, Szego T, et al. Intra-operative transgastric ERCP after a Roux-en-Y gastric bypass. Endoscopy 2007;39:E219–20.
29. Patel JA, Patel NA, Shinde T, et al. Endoscopic retrograde cholangiopancreatography after laparoscopic Roux-en-Y gastric bypass: a case series and review of the literature. Am Surg 2008;74:689–93.
30. Mutignani M, Marchese M, Tringali A, et al. Laparoscopy-assisted ERCP after biliopancreatic diversion. Obes Surg 2007;17:251–4.
31. Roberts KF, Panait L, Duffy AJ, et al. Laparoscopic-assisted transgastric endoscopy: current indications and future implications. JSLS 2008;12:30–6.
32. Lopes TL, Clements RH, Wilcox CM. Laparoscopic-assisted ERCP: experience from a high volume bariatric surgery center. Gastrointest Endosc 2009;70: 1254–9.
33. Carmody B, DeMaria EJ, Johnson JM, et al. Internal hernia after laparoscopic Roux-en-Y gastric bypass. Surg Obes Relat Dis 2005;1:511–6.
34. Cho M, Pinto D, Carrodeguas L, et al. Frequency and management of internal hernias after laparoscopic antecolic antegastric Roux-en-Y gastric bypass without division of the small bowel mesentery or closure of mesenteric defects: review of 1400 consecutive cases. Surg Obes Relat Dis 2006;2:87–91.

Postoperative Metabolic and Nutritional Complications of Bariatric Surgery

Timothy R. Koch, MD[a,b,*], Frederick C. Finelli, MD, JD[c,d]

KEYWORDS

- Micronutient • Malnutrition • Bariatric surgery
- Diabetes mellitus

In the majority of patients with medically complicated obesity (commonly termed "morbid obesity"), it is difficult to effectively treat obesity by the combination of a pharmacologic agent, dietary changes, and exercise. Surgery to reduce and control weight has therefore become an important technique. After undergoing bariatric surgery, both macronutrient (such as protein) and micronutrient deficiencies are common. The type of bariatric surgery is important in understanding the potential risk of developing postoperative nutritional disorders. The rising risk of developing nutritional disorders following different types of bariatric surgery is: laparoscopic adjustable gastric banding < vertical sleeve gastrectomy < divided Roux-en-Y gastric bypass < bilio-pancreatic diversion.

In the performance of a laparoscopic adjustable gastric banding, the surgical dissection is designed to make a small pouch below the gastroesophageal junction but to keep the band above the peritoneal reflection of the lesser sac with a tunnel made through the retro-gastric attachments. The band is introduced and the tunnel

[a] Georgetown University School of Medicine, 3900 Reservoir Road, NW, Washington, DC 20057, USA
[b] Department of Surgery, Washington Hospital Center, 110 Irving Street, NW, Washington, DC 20010, USA
[c] Department of Surgery, Washington Hospital Center, #3400 North, 106 Irving Street, NW, Washington, DC 20010, USA
[d] Performance Improvement and Safety, Washington Hospital Center, 110 Irving Street, NW, Washington, DC 20010, USA
* Corresponding author. Department of Surgery, Washington Hospital Center, 110 Irving Street, NW, Washington, DC 20010.
E-mail address: timothy.r.koch@medstar.net (T.R. Koch).

Gastroenterol Clin N Am 39 (2010) 109–124
doi:10.1016/j.gtc.2009.12.003
0889-8553/10/$ – see front matter © 2010 Elsevier Inc. All rights reserved.

gastro.theclinics.com

aids in prevention of band migration. Band adjustment is deferred at the time of surgery and the injection reservoir is attached by tubing to the band and is implanted on the anterior rectus sheath. There are few long-term studies of the nutritional consequences of this surgery. As in any intervention that induces weight loss, vitamin D deficiency must be periodically excluded.

In the surgical construction of a restrictive vertical sleeve gastrectomy (gastric sleeve resection), multiple staplers are used to produce a tubular gastric pouch through resection of 60% to 80% of the stomach along the greater curvature. For greater weight loss, this procedure can be combined with a second malabsorptive procedure, the duodenal switch. In a duodenal switch, the duodenum is transected 5 cm distal to the pylorus and the distal duodenal segment (stump) is oversewn. The small intestine is then transected approximately one-third of its length to the ileocecal valve; the distal transected segment is used to produce an anastomosis to proximal duodenum, while the proximal transected segment is used to produce an entero-enteric anastomosis 75 to 100 cm proximal to the ileocecal valve.

The most commonly performed bariatric surgical procedure in the United States is the divided Roux-en-Y gastric bypass (**Fig. 1**). This procedure combines restriction of food intake, due to the small size of the gastric pouch (≤30 mL) and constriction at the gastrojejunal anastomosis (10–13 mm diameter), with malabsorption induced by bypass of the duodenum and proximal jejunum. In an extended gastric bypass, the entero-enteric anastomosis is formed 120 cm or less from the ileocecal valve. Classic studies of the Roux-en-Y reconstruction performed by Chey and colleagues[1] demonstrated malabsorption of both fat and nitrogen. Malabsorption of fat and protein was correctable by providing exogenous pancreatic enzymes. However, these findings were not clinically significant in this group of patients (who had undergone surgical

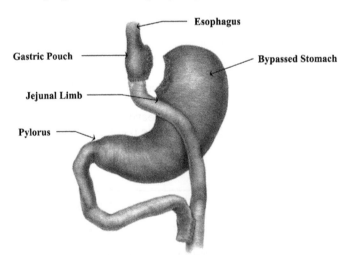

Fig. 1. Divided Roux-en-Y gastric bypass surgery. The surgeon produces a gastric pouch of less than 1 ounce (30 mL). The jejunum is divided 30 to 70 cm distal to the native duodeno-jejunal junction. Exclusion of the stomach, duodenum, and proximal jejunum alters absorption of vitamin B12, iron, and thiamine. Nutritional disorders can result from the length of the common channel, which extends from the jejuno-jejunal anastomosis to the ileocecal valve. A short common channel (≤120 cm), as is formed in a bilio-pancreatic diversion, will induce a more severe malabsorptive disorder. (*Reproduced from* Lakhani SV, Shah HN, Alexander K, et al. Small intestinal bacterial overgrowth and thiamine deficiency after Roux-en-Y gastric bypass surgery in obese patients. Nutr Res 2008;28(5):293–8; with permission.)

therapy for ulcer disease) because the patients were able to increase their daily caloric intake. The findings emphasize the importance in performance of the Roux-en-Y gastric bypass of restriction of food intake by combining a small gastric pouch with constriction at the gastrojejunal anastomosis.

The major feature of a bilio-pancreatic diversion in a duodenal switch or in an extended Roux-en-Y gastric bypass is that the entero-enteric anastomosis is formed 120 cm or less from the ileocecal valve to induce a significant malabsorption. The distance from the entero-enteric anastomosis to the ileocecal valve is called the "common channel." The malabsorptive disorder induced by a short common channel ($\leq$120 cm) is in part due to bile salt malabsorption with, consequently, secondary steathorrhea. Bilio-pancreatic diversion induces more severe deficiencies of fat-soluble vitamins as well as essential fatty acid deficiencies.

METABOLIC CONSEQUENCES OF BARIATRIC SURGERY
Metabolic Syndrome

The medical management of patients who have developed metabolic syndrome is a major health care issue in the United States. The complexity of this chronic disorder leads to joint patient management by multiple medical specialists. The prevalence of metabolic syndrome has risen, and there is a direct relationship to the increase in prevalence of medically complicated obesity.[2]

The potential for bariatric surgery to be used as a primary therapy for metabolic syndrome has been a focus in clinical studies. In a study from the Mayo Clinic of patients who underwent Roux-en-Y gastric bypass compared with patients treated with a medical management program, metabolic syndrome was defined by standard components: increased blood triglycerides, low high-density lipoprotein, hypertension, hyperglycemia, and obesity.[3] After a mean follow-up of 3.4 years, patients treated with a medical management program had only a significant decrease in high-density lipoprotein levels, whereas patients who had undergone bariatric surgery were found to have significant declines in all components of the metabolic syndrome. With the use of a medical management program, there was only a 12% decline in the number of patients with metabolic syndrome, whereas in patients who underwent bariatric surgery there was a 66% decline. This study provides strong evidence for the superiority of Roux-en-Y gastric bypass for the long-term management of patients with the metabolic syndrome.

Regulation of Insulin Secretion

The next major question regarding the metabolic consequences of bariatric surgery is centered on the mechanisms by which bariatric surgery improves control of diabetes mellitus. Understanding these mechanisms could improve clinical decision making in the process of recommending a specific bariatric surgical procedure to an individual patient.

It has been known for many years that patients who underwent Roux-en-Y gastric bypass had major improvements in their hyperglycemia even before major weight loss had occurred. The potential role of gut endocrine peptides that alter insulin secretion by the pancreas has been considered. Incretins are insulinotrophic gut-derived hormones. Major incretins in the gut-pancreas axis include glucose-dependent insulinotrophic polypeptide (GIP), which is released from the duodenum and proximal jejunum in response to intake of glucose and fat, and glucagons-like peptide-1 (GLP-1), which is produced by posttranslational processing of preproglucagon. Endocrine cells in the gut that secrete preproglucagon are the same endocrine cells that secrete peptide YY, which the authors have shown are present in highest concentrations in the ileum and colon.[4] Both GIP and GLP-1 affect pancreatic β-cell function.[5]

Studies of incretin secretion after bariatric surgery support increased insulin secretion induced by nutrient-mediated secretion of incretins in patients who have undergone Roux-en-Y gastric bypass, whereas a normalization of insulin resistance has been observed after bilio-pancreatic diversion, a more malabsorptive bariatric procedure.[6] However, a recent study did compare Roux-en-Y gastric bypass surgery with sleeve gastrectomy.[7] This study identified increased postprandial insulin and GLP-1 levels after both bariatric surgical procedures, and both bariatric procedures had similar insulin and GLP-1 secretion after 3 months.[7] These findings suggest that bypass of the proximal small intestine in patients who undergo Roux-en-Y gastric bypass is not the sole mechanism to explain altered secretion of incretins.

There have also been studies that compare Roux-en-Y gastric bypass with adjustable gastric banding.[8,9] These studies have supported the role of increased postprandial secretion of the incretin, GLP-1, at up to 1 year after Roux-en-Y gastric bypass but not after adjustable gastric banding. Improved fasting glucose control in patients after adjustable gastric banding seems to be related to weight loss and increased insulin levels, with no apparent relationship to incretin levels.

Control of Hyperglycemia

The use of bariatric surgery for treatment of diabetes mellitus includes at least 2 major clinical issues. The first major issue is whether bariatric surgery is a first-line treatment for medically complicated obesity in those patients who have poor control of hyperglycemia. The second, which is now being examined, is whether bariatric surgery might prevent or reverse development of complications of diabetes mellitus in patients who have adequate therapy thus preventing hyperglycemia.

In studies of patients who have undergone bariatric surgery, 87% of patients with type 2 diabetes mellitus develop improvement or resolution of their disease postoperatively.[10] The greatest weight loss and resolution of diabetes mellitus has been seen in patients who have undergone bilio-pancreatic diversion or Roux-en-Y gastric bypass, whereas after adjustable gastric banding a smaller percentage of patients have resolution of diabetes mellitus.[10] Suggested explanations for this marked clinical improvement after Roux-en-Y gastric bypass include increased insulin secretion in the immediate postoperative period, but decreased peripheral insulin sensitivity 6 months after bariatric surgery.[11] Other investigators have favored weight loss as being the major factor in the development of remission of type 2 diabetes mellitus after Roux-en-Y gastric bypass[12] although, as previously mentioned, it is a common clinical observation that patients have a significant decline in their therapy requirements for diabetes mellitus immediately after Roux-en-Y gastric bypass.

Patients can develop improved control of hyperglycemia after adjustable gastric banding, a restrictive bariatric surgical procedure. It has been reported that patients after adjustable gastric banding have reduced peripheral insulin resistance 6 months after surgery, with no changes in insulin secretion.[11] In a separate study, 73% of patients who underwent adjustable gastric banding achieved remission of type 2 diabetes mellitus at 2 years, compared with only 13% in a separate control group of patients who were treated with conventional diabetes care with a focus on weight loss by lifestyle changes.[13] In this study, it was suggested that remission of type 2 diabetes mellitus was related to weight loss in those patients who underwent adjustable gastric banding.[13]

Hyperinsulinemic Hypoglycemia

A small group of patients present with complaints of dizziness, syncope, or near-syncope following Roux-en-Y gastric bypass surgery. A diagnosis of hypoglycemia must be considered, but may be difficult to identify. Recent work has supported the presence of hyperinsulinemia in response to oral glucose in Roux-en-Y gastric bypass, both in patients who are symptomatic as well as in those who are asymptomatic.[14] This finding supports the notion that hyperinsulinemia is the result of Roux-en-Y gastric bypass.

Standard medical management has included dietary recommendations for restriction of intake of simple sugars. Patients have been instructed to carry a supplement with high simple sugar content with them for intake if a symptom develops. A select group of high-risk patients in the United States have undergone pancreatectomy with successful management of this disorder. Medical managements of this disorder with the use of diazoxide[15] or with a combination of verapamil and acarbose[16] have been described in case reports.

MACRONUTRIENTS
Protein Deficiency

In weight reduction protocols, postoperative bariatric patients are instructed to maintain intake of 60 to 70 g of protein daily. Although it can occur after Roux-en-Y gastric bypass, significant protein malabsorption is most likely after a bilio-pancreatic diversion, in which protein malabsorption increases the risk of developing protein malnutrition.

Monitoring of patients can be difficult. It has been shown that serum albumin concentrations cannot discriminate between well and undernourished patients.[17,18] In patients who present with hypoalbuminemia, it is important to consider inflammatory processes such as small intestinal bacterial overgrowth as the source.[19] In monitoring a patient's response to nutritional therapy, a shorter half-life protein such as prealbumin may be followed over time.

Hair loss is a common early clinical manifestation of postoperative protein malnutrition (alopecia can also occur during zinc deficiency). Long-term manifestations of protein malnutrition can include muscle mass wasting and edema; a protein deficiency similar to Kwashiorkor has been described after Roux-en-Y gastric bypass.[20]

MICRONUTRIENTS

Micronutrients that are essential dietary factors are those nutrients that cannot be synthesized by humans. Specific micronutrients are required in micro- or milligram quantities in a diverse array of biochemical pathways and metabolic processes. These micronutrients include water-soluble and fat-soluble vitamins, and trace elements. Vitamins are subdivided into 2 groups, fat-soluble vitamins (vitamins A, D, E, and K) and water-soluble vitamins.

A significant deficiency of an essential micronutrient can induce a clinical syndrome. One recent survey has reported an increased risk during the first 1 year after bariatric surgery of development of vitamin A, vitamin D, and thiamine deficiency.[21] A second recent survey has reported that the prevalence 1 year after bariatric surgery of elevated homocysteine levels is 29%, low ferritin is 15%, low vitamin B12 is 11%, low red blood cell folate is 12%, and vitamin D deficiency is 57%.[22] A twice-daily chewable multivitamin is recommended after a malabsorptive, bariatric surgery (**Box 1**), and a once-daily chewable multivitamin is recommended after laparoscopic adjustable gastric banding or a vertical sleeve gastrectomy. Daily calcium supplements are recommended for all patients after bariatric surgery (see **Box 1**).

Box 1
Vitamin and mineral supplements after malabsorptive bariatric surgery

1. MULTIVITAMIN with MINERALS: 1 chewable tablet, daily to twice a day

2. CALCIUM SUPPLEMENTS: chewable tablets, 1.2 g elemental calcium, daily

Specific deficiencies

3. THIAMINE: 100 mg tablet, twice daily or THIAMINE: 100–250 mg intramuscular, monthly

4. NIACIN: 500 mg orally, 3 times daily

5. FOLIC ACID: 1–5 mg orally, daily

6. VITAMIN B12: 1000 μg, intramuscular, monthly or SUBLINGUAL VITAMIN B12: 500 μg tablet once daily

7. VITAMIN A: 10,000 IU orally, daily

8. VITAMIN D (ergocalciferol): 50,000 IU with a meal once weekly (up to 12 weeks) followed by VITAMIN D3 (cholecalciferol): 1000 IU with a meal twice daily

9. VITAMIN E: 800–1200 IU orally, daily

10. VITAMIN K: 5–20 mg orally, daily

11. IRON: iron/vitamin C complex, 1 tablet daily before a meal, iron elixir (through a straw), or parenteral iron

12. ZINC SULFATE: 220 mg capsule, daily to every other day

13. COPPER GLUCONATE: 2 mg capsule, daily to every other day

FAT-SOLUBLE VITAMINS
Vitamin A

Vitamin A complex includes retinols, β-carotenes, and carotenoids. The human liver generally stores a 1-year supply of vitamin A. When ingested in high doses either acutely or chronically, vitamin A may cause toxic manifestations, including headache, vomiting, diplopia, alopecia, dryness of the mucous membranes, bone abnormalities, and liver damage. Signs of toxicity usually appear with sustained daily intakes exceeding 15,000 IU. As an alternative supplement, signs of toxicity have not been observed while receiving β-carotene, the pre-vitamin A analogue.

Vitamin A deficiency after bariatric surgery is most commonly seen in patients who have undergone a bilio-pancreatic diversion, duodenal switch, or extended Roux-en-Y gastric bypass. In these procedures, the mechanism of deficiency is most likely related to fat-soluble vitamin malabsorption induced by bile acid deficiency. In addition, individuals with zinc deficiency have impaired protein synthesis that may alter retinol transport from the liver to other organs. Common manifestations of vitamin A deficiency include nocturnal visual difficulty, dry skin, dry hair, and pruritus. Other potential manifestations include decreased visual acuity and reduced resistance to infections. Treatment of vitamin A deficiency includes supplemental vitamin A, 10,000 IU daily by mouth (see **Box 1**) as well as cotherapy for any existing iron deficiency, because vitamin A deficiency may persist in the presence of iron deficiency.

Vitamin D

It is important to simultaneously consider the potential for vitamin D deficiency and calcium malabsorption because vitamin D deficiency activates a metabolic cascade resulting in hypocalcemia, secondary hyperparathyroidism, and subsequently osteoporosis and osteomalacia.[23,24] Isolated serum calcium measurement is not an adequate marker of calcium metabolism. Patients may present clinically with complaints of bony pain, back pain, or aching of the limbs.

Multiple explanations have been proposed for vitamin D deficiency. First, it has been reported that a large percentage of patients with medically complicated obesity have vitamin D deficiency.[22] In addition, vitamin D malabsorption results from bile salt deficiency, especially in those patients who have undergone a bilio-pancreatic diversion during bariatric surgery. Patients who have a rapid weight loss phase from any cause require additional vitamin D. Finally, preliminary studies suggest that small intestinal bacterial overgrowth interferes with vitamin D absorption.

In preliminary studies, bariatric surgery patients maintain normal serum calcium by decreasing urinary calcium secretion. Urine calcium secretion can, however, be altered by concomitant use of diuretics. It is therefore important to monitor total 25-hydroxyvitamin D levels, 24-hour urinary calcium, and serum alkaline phosphatase at least every 6 months postoperatively. Parathyroid hormone determination and dual energy x-ray absorptiometry scan should be considered in patients who have prolonged or difficult to treat vitamin D deficiency and elevation of the bone fraction of serum alkaline phosphatase. A patient with an elevation of the parathyroid hormone level requires additional supplementation with vitamin D and calcium.

It is recommended that all patients after bariatric surgery use daily supplements to include at least 1.2 g daily of elemental calcium and 800 international units of vitamin D (see **Box 1**). Patients with low serum levels of 25-hydroxyvitamin D are treated initially with 50,000 IU of vitamin D (ergocalciferol) orally once per week for 6 to 8 weeks (see **Box 1**). A recheck of 25-hydroxyvitamin D level after 8 weeks is recommended to confirm repletion.[25] The reported dose for treatment of rickets is at least 600,000 IU. Treatment of up to 150,000 IU taken 4 times, during 1 day of treatment has been described, although the authors generally provide 50,000 IU taken daily with a meal for 12 days, because of anecdotal reports of liver test abnormalities associated with high-dose oral vitamin D.

Vitamin E

Vitamin E consists of tocopherols and tocotrienols. This fat-soluble vitamin, once absorbed, is located in cell membranes where it is thought to be active in preventing lipid peroxidation. Most adults seem to tolerate doses of vitamin E alone up to 1000 mg per day (0.67 mg of vitamin E is 1 IU) without gross signs or biochemical evidence of toxicity.[26]

Deficiency of vitamin E should be considered in individuals who have visual symptoms (retinopathy), nonspecific neurologic symptoms (ataxia, loss of vibration and position sensation, muscle weakness, or ptosis), or hemolytic anemia. Treatment of vitamin E deficiency should include oral vitamin E 800 to 1200 IU daily (see **Box 1**).

Vitamin K

Vitamin K is the name given to a group of compounds, all of which contain the 2-methyl-1,4-naphthoquinone moiety. These compounds are essential for the formation of prothrombin, and 5 factors (factors VII, IX, and X, and proteins C and S) that are involved in regulation of blood clotting. Under normal conditions, vitamin K is moderately (40%–70%) well absorbed from the jejunum and ileum, but very poorly absorbed in the colon.[27]

Absorption of vitamin K and other lipid-soluble vitamins depends on the normal flow of bile and pancreatic secretion, and is enhanced by dietary fat. The total body pool of vitamin K is small and its turnover is rapid. Most of the daily requirements for vitamin K is provided through its biosynthesis by the intestinal flora. Deficiency of vitamin K leads to increase risk of bleeding disorders. Replacement of vitamin K can be obtained either with an oral form (5–20 mg daily) (see **Box 1**) or with parenteral delivery of the vitamin.

WATER-SOLUBLE VITAMINS

The biochemical roles of water-soluble vitamins and the associated deficiency disorders are shown in **Table 1**. There are only minor stores of water-soluble vitamins in the body.

Thiamine

Thiamine or vitamin B1 deficiency is a major nutritional complication following Roux-en-Y gastric bypass surgery, and is common in the patient population.[28] Thiamine deficiency (beriberi) was originally described in individuals with multiorgan involvement, including cardiac, gastrointestinal, or neuropsychiatric symptoms that corrected with "beriberi factor" (thiamine or vitamin B1). The authors have described the presence of thiamine deficiency that does not correct with oral thiamine in patients who have undergone Roux-en-Y gastric bypass.[28] "Bariatric beriberi" is associated with small intestinal bacterial overgrowth, and concomitant antibiotic therapy is required to correct thiamine deficiency.[28]

Among the major clinical presentations of beriberi (**Table 2**), patients with neuropsychiatric beriberi may have auditory and visual hallucinations, or aggressive behavior. Wernicke disease presents with confusion (impairment of memory or altered mental state), nystagmus, ataxia, and ophthalmoplegia. Patients with high-output cardiovascular disease (wet beriberi) have been reported to have tachycardia, respiratory distress, or lower extremity edema, with right-to-left ventricular dilation and lactic acidosis. Patients with neurologic (dry beriberi) are seen with numbness or muscle weakness, pain of lower to upper extremities, or convulsions. These patients may have exaggerated tendon reflexes. Gastrointestinal beriberi induces delayed emptying of the stomach. After gastric bypass surgery, common symptoms include nausea and emesis in patients with megajejunum, and constipation in patients with megacolon.

In laboratory confirmation of the diagnosis, it is known that only a small percentage of total body thiamine is present in whole blood. An alternative approach to support a diagnosis of thiamine deficiency is measurement of erythrocyte transketolase

Table 1
Water-soluble vitamins as coenzyme precursors and deficiency disorders

Vitamin	Coenzyme Derivative	Deficiency Disorders
Thiamine (vitamin B1)	Thiamine pyrophosphate (TPP)	Beriberi
Riboflavin (vitamin B2)	Flavin adenine dinucleotide (FAD)	Eye disorders, glossitis, dermatitis
Niacin (nicotinic acid)	Nicotinamide adenine dinucleotide	Pellagra
Folate	Tetrahydrofolate	Macrocytic anemia
Biotin	Pyruvate carboxylase	
Pantothenic acid	Coenzyme A	
Pyridoxine (vitamin B6)	Pyridoxal phosphate	Dermatitis
Vitamin B12	5'-Deoxyadenosyl-cobalamine	Neuropathy, anemia

Table 2
Clinical presentations of thiamine deficiency

Beriberi Subtype	Symptoms and Findings
Neuropsychiatric	Hallucinations/aggressive behavior Confusion/nystagmus/ataxia/ophthalmoplegia
Wet beriberi	Tachycardia/respiratory distress/leg edema Right ventricular dilation/lactic acidosis
Dry beriberi	Numbness/muscle weakness and pain of lower to upper extremities/ convulsions Exaggerated tendon reflexes
Gastrointestinal	Nausea/emesis and megajejunum Constipation and megacolon
Bariatric beriberi	Symptoms corrected by antibiotics, not by oral thiamine

activity.[29] This bioassay is based on biochemical evidence that the catalytic activity of the enzyme transketolase depends on its binding to thiamine pyrophosphate.

Acute psychosis and Wernicke encephalopathy are medical emergencies. These conditions require hospitalization with supportive care and a minimum of 250 mg of thiamine given daily, intramuscularly or intravenously infused over 3 to 4 hours (to reduce the risk of an anaphylactoid reaction) for at least 3 to 5 days.[30]

The standard therapy for thiamine deficiency is thiamine HCl, 100 mg, taken orally twice daily (see **Box 1**). In patients who do not respond to oral thiamine, the presence of small intestinal bacterial overgrowth must be considered. A diagnosis of small intestinal bacterial overgrowth is supported by elevation of serum folate level or by a rapid increase in breath hydrogen or methane following an oral dose of glucose.[28] In patients with symptoms suggesting beriberi, thiamine HCl, 100 to 250 mg, should be given intramuscularly. Most patients report symptomatic improvement within several days after the first parenteral dose of thiamine HCl. The clinician must then determine whether the patient can prevent symptom recurrence with use of oral thiamine, or whether intermittent parenteral thiamine will be required.

Riboflavin

Even though only small stores of riboflavin are present in the body, its deficiency has not been specifically reported after bariatric surgery. Vitamin B2 is present in the flavocoenzymes, flavin adenine dinucleotide, and flavin mononucleotide. Flavocoenzymes are a major participant in several reactions important in metabolic pathways and in the proper functioning of glutathione peroxidase (required for metabolism of hydroperoxides) as well as glutathione reductase (generates reduced glutathione from oxidized glutathione). Studies by the authors have shown in a mouse model that deficiency of reduced glutathione induces an enterocolitis mimicking the appearance of Crohn disease.[31] Clinical symptoms of riboflavin deficiency include sore throat, stomatitis, anemia, and a scaly dermatitis.

Niacin

Deficiency of niacin has not been evaluated and reported after bariatric surgery. It is difficult to diagnose niacin deficiency by laboratory studies, but the diagnosis is supported by low plasma niacin. Nicotinic acid or vitamin B3 is converted into nicotinamide, a component of nicotinamide adenine dinucleotide (involved in catabolic reactions) and nicotinamide adenine dinucleotide phosphate (involved in anabolic reactions). Severe deficiency of niacin is termed pellagra and includes neurologic, dermatologic, and gastrointestinal involvement. Clinical manifestations to be considered include headaches, ataxia or myoclonus, anxiety-depression, delusions or hallucinations, painful, scaly dermatitis, and a malabsorptive disorder or diarrhea with colitis. The basic treatment of pellagra (see **Box 1**) is initiation of oral niacin, 500 mg, 3 times daily (this may induce flushing).

Folate

Folate levels in patients after Roux-en-Y gastric bypass surgery must be considered in the context of the patient's risk for small intestinal bacterial overgrowth. In studies of small intestinal bacterial overgrowth, a high serum folate level is an identified and validated marker for bacterial overgrowth.[32,33] In the detection of small intestinal bacterial overgrowth, it is known that the finding of high serum folate has a good specificity (79%) but only a low sensitivity (51%).

In patients who have folate deficiency after bariatric surgery, one should consider the potential for another small intestinal malabsorptive disorder, including celiac sprue. Patients with folate deficiency are generally detected in this patient population in individuals with a normocytic, mixed anemia with an increased red cell distribution width. Treatment of folate deficiency includes oral folic acid, 1 to 5 mg daily (see **Box 1**).

Vitamin B12

Vitamin B12 deficiency is a well-described nutritional deficiency after bariatric surgery[34] and likely involves a multifactorial origin. Roux-en-Y gastric bypass results in the exclusion of the majority of parietal cell mass, which is a site of R factor and intrinsic factor production. In addition, relative achlorhydria after bariatric surgery prevents oral cyanocobalamin from being deconjugated from pteryl groups before absorption of cyanocobalamin. A final potential mechanism of vitamin B12 deficiency is utility of this substance by overgrowth of bacteria in the proximal small intestine.

Because of storage of vitamin B12, development of vitamin B12 deficiency may manifest several years after bariatric surgery. Classic clinical manifestations are the multiple presentations of pernicious anemia or development of peripheral neuropathy. A low normal blood level of vitamin B12 can indicate the presence of deficiency. Confirmation of vitamin B12 deficiency is supported by finding an increased serum level of methylmalonic acid.[35]

In the treatment of vitamin B12 deficiency, daily, oral cobalamin is considered less effective than the intramuscular preparation.[34] Treatment of vitamin B12 deficiency (see **Box 1**) includes oral vitamin B12 (cyanocobalamin) 350 to 500 µg per day, intramuscular vitamin B12 1000 µg every month or 3000 µg every 6 months, or a nasal (500 µg once weekly) or sublingual (500 µg once daily) preparation that is absorbed locally.

TRACE ELEMENTS

Trace elements function as cofactors for antioxidant enzymes or proteins (**Table 3**). Trace elements in supplements provide a relatively narrow range of safety between deficiency and toxicity. Because of their ability to donate or accept electrons, transition metals have potential antioxidant properties. Three key metals that have been examined as antioxidants are zinc, selenium, and iron.

Table 3
Trace elements as cofactors for enzymes/proteins and associated deficiency disorders

Element	Enzymes/Proteins	Deficiency Disorders
Copper	Cytochrome oxidases Cytosolic superoxide dismutase	Anemia, neutropenia Myelopathy
Zinc	Cytosolic superoxide dismutase	Dermatitis, alopecia, glossitis, nail dystrophy
Manganese	Mitochondrial superoxide dismutase	
Selenium	Glutathione peroxidase	Cardiomyopathy
Iron	Catalase/hemoglobin	Anemia

Zinc

Zinc has a role as a cellular antioxidant.[36] One of the ways in which zinc functions is via induction of metallothioneins, a group of low molecular weight amino acid residues. Production of metallothioneins is induced by zinc in the liver, gut, and kidney. Metallothioneins have been shown to scavenge free radicals and bind some oxidants.[36,37] Zinc has also been shown to regulate the levels of the extracellular form of superoxide dismutase (SOD).[38] Zinc may reduce the formation of the highly toxic hydroxyradical (OH^-) from H_2O_2 produced through the antagonism of redox-active transition metals, such as iron and copper.[36]

Zinc deficiency in bariatric patients has not been well studied. Symptoms of zinc deficiency include a dermatologic eruption, alopecia, glossitis, and nail dystrophy.[39] Treatment of zinc deficiency is with oral zinc sulfate, 220 mg capsule, taken daily to every other day (see **Box 1**).

Selenium

Selenium is a trace element that is known to be essential for activation of glutathione peroxidase, a key enzyme in the body's defense against oxygen-derived free radicals. For this reason selenium supplementation, alone and in combination with other micronutrients, has been extensively studied. It has been suggested that selenium toxicity, which primarily affects the immune system, may be limited to inorganic rather than the organic forms of this trace element.[40] Selenium deficiency induces a cardiomyopathy in those regions of the world in which selenium levels in the soil are low.

Iron

After bariatric surgery, many patients require iron supplementation to treat anemia. There are multiple potential mechanisms that may explain iron malabsorption after bariatric surgery, including a relatively achlorhydric gastric pouch (acid may improve absorption of nonheme iron from plant sources) and bypass of the duodenum and proximal jejunum (the major locations of iron absorption). Identification of iron deficiency in a bariatric patient requires consideration of other origins for anemia such as colon cancer, gastric or esophageal cancer, celiac sprue, and so forth. Patients with normal hemoglobin levels can have low ferritin levels postoperatively, supporting the addition of iron supplementation. Routine treatment of iron deficiency (see **Box 1**) includes treatment with an iron/vitamin C complex or with 150 to 200 mg per day of oral elemental iron in any preparation (gluconate/sulfate/fumarate) as is best tolerated by the patient. Parenteral iron is occasionally needed in those patients who have a poor response to oral iron therapy, especially in premenopausal women with heavy menstrual bleeding.

It is rarely recognized that iron supplementation has some risks. Catalase, the enzyme that catalyzes the decomposition of hydrogen peroxide, is a hemeprotein. Iron supplementation for whatever purpose should be monitored, because electron transfer from transition metals such as iron to oxygen-containing molecules can initiate free radical reactions. Large doses of unnecessary iron supplements could induce an acquired iron overload.

Copper

There is a joint transport mechanism for the micronutrients copper and zinc.[41] High-dose zinc intake can therefore induce copper deficiency. Liquid vitamin supplements may be deficient in copper. The occurrence of copper deficiency has been reported in patients after Roux-en-Y gastric bypass.[42] Copper deficiency induces hematological (anemia and neutropenia) and neurologic (myelopathy presenting with spastic gait and sensory ataxia) manifestations.[43] In patients with copper deficiency, clinical and neuroimaging findings mimic the findings seen in patients with deficiency of vitamin B12.[43] Treatment of copper deficiency is with oral copper gluconate, 2 mg capsule, taken daily to every other day (see **Box 1**). Oral supplementation, however, may not fully correct copper deficiency.

NUTRITIONAL CONSEQUENCES OF BARIATRIC SURGERY

Periodic laboratory testing is recommended for all patients after malabsorptive bariatric surgery, as summarized in **Table 4**. It is not presently known whether routine laboratory testing prevents the development of a complication after bariatric surgery. Therefore, a reasonable medical approach is to reevaluate patients on a regular schedule (see **Table 4**) after bariatric surgery to exclude development of specific postoperative nutritional disorders, as summarized in the following.

Anemia

In patients who have undergone a malabsorptive bariatric procedure, anemia is a common postoperative finding. Microcytic anemia supports the presence of iron deficiency, and the presence of macrocytic anemia raises the question of deficiency of vitamin B12 or folate.

Persistent iron deficiency anemia despite oral supplementation with iron supports consideration of iron loss from a colon source, from a stomal ulcer, or from the excluded pancreaticobiliary limb (duodenal ulcer or gastric ulcer/antritis in the

Table 4 Routine laboratory testing after malabsorptive bariatric surgery	
Interval	**Laboratory Testing**
3 months postoperatively	Complete blood count; glucose; glycosylated hemoglobin[a]; lipids; chemistry group
At 6-month intervals during first 3 years & then once yearly	Chemistry group; complete blood count; lipids; ferritin; zinc; copper; magnesium; vitamin A; total 25-hydroxy vitamin D; folate; whole blood thiamine; vitamin B12; 24-hour urinary calcium

[a] If diabetes mellitus is present preoperatively.

excluded stomach). Refractory iron deficiency may require parenteral iron (often seen in premenopausal women with menses).

Anemia following bariatric surgery that is not corrected by iron or vitamin B12 supplementation is a complex disorder.[44,45] Vitamin E deficiency can induce a hemolytic anemia. Copper deficiency can result in anemia and neutropenia. In addition to addressing the question of potential blood loss from the gastric remnant or the small intestine, the authors exclude other nutritional origins of anemia by examining blood levels of vitamin A, vitamin E, folate, zinc, and copper (**Table 5**).

Neurologic Disorders

After malabsorptive bariatric surgery, peripheral neuropathy is the most common neurologic symptom.[46] Neurologic complaints are reported by 1.3% to 4.6% of postoperative patients in surveys.[46] Reported neurologic emergencies include Wernicke encephalopathy (thiamine deficiency) and Guillain-Barré syndrome.[46]

Thiamine deficiency can result in a group of neurologic symptoms including numbness, muscle weakness, extremity pain, or convulsions in dry beriberi; auditory hallucinations, visual hallucinations, or aggressive behavior in neuropsychiatric beriberi; and confusion, nystagmus, ataxia, or ophthalmoplegia in Wernicke disease. In patients with niacin deficiency (pellagra), neurologic manifestations include headaches, ataxia or myoclonus, anxiety-depression, delusions, or hallucinations. Vitamin E deficiency should be considered in individuals who have neurologic symptoms of ataxia, loss of vibration and position sensation, muscle weakness, or ptosis, whereas vitamin B12 deficiency can present with evidence for a peripheral neuropathy. Copper deficiency induces a myelopathy (with spastic gait and sensory ataxia), and the clinical and neuroimaging findings in copper deficiency mimic the findings of vitamin B12 deficiency.[43]

In the authors' experience, patients may have ophthalmologic or peripheral neurologic symptoms that have not been reported to their primary care provider. In patients with neurologic symptoms, the authors obtain blood levels of niacin, vitamin B12, vitamin E, copper, and a whole blood thiamine (see **Table 5**).

Visual Disorders

Manifestations of vitamin A deficiency include nocturnal visual difficulty and decreased visual acuity, whereas vitamin E deficiency can induce visual symptoms related to retinopathy. Patients with thiamine deficiency can present with complaints of difficulty focusing their vision or persistent blurred vision; on physical examination, nystagmus is often identified. In laboratory evaluation, the authors obtain blood levels of vitamin A, vitamin E, and whole blood thiamine (see **Table 5**).

Table 5	
Laboratory testing for nutritional disorders after bariatric surgery	
Disorder	**Laboratory Blood Tests**
Anemia	Ferritin; vitamin B12; folate & then consider vitamin A; vitamin E; zinc; copper
Neurologic disorders	Vitamin B12; whole blood thiamine & then consider vitamin E; copper; plasma niacin
Visual disorders	Vitamin A; vitamin E; whole blood thiamine
Skin disorders	Vitamin A; zinc; plasma niacin
Edema	Selenium; whole blood thiamine; plasma niacin

Skin Disorders

Manifestations of vitamin A deficiency include xerosis and pruritus. Essential fatty acid deficiency, niacin deficiency, and riboflavin deficiency can cause a scaly dermatitis. The essential fatty acids linoleic acid and linolenic acid are both present in flaxseed oil, soybean oil, and canola oil. Symptoms of zinc deficiency include a dermatologic eruption. The authors obtain blood levels of vitamin A, niacin, and zinc (see **Table 5**).

Edema

Underlying heart failure is a major consideration when a patient presents with edema. Patients with thiamine deficiency can develop high-output cardiovascular disease (wet beriberi) and have been reported to have tachycardia, respiratory distress, or lower extremity edema, with right-to-left ventricular dilation and lactic acidosis. Selenium deficiency is another known cause of heart failure. From a patient with edema the authors obtain blood selenium, whole blood thiamine, and plasma niacin (see **Table 5**).

Edema can develop in patients with hypoalbuminemia. An underlying hepatic disorder, potentially the end result of steatohepatitis, should be considered. Other origins of hypoalbuminemia include an inflammatory process and small intestinal bacterial overgrowth. There is a serious syndrome of postoperative diarrhea associated with hypoalbuminenia and diffuse edema. There are several considerations. This disorder may be induced by severe protein/calorie malnutrition due to a biliopancreatic diversion such as an extended (distal) Roux-en-Y gastric bypass or a duodenal switch, because both procedures can result in severe steatorrhea/malabsorption. In addition, it has been reported that this syndrome improves with antibiotic therapy,[19] supporting the role of small intestinal bacterial overgrowth. Finally, niacin deficiency can induce a diarrheal illness or colitis that may be responsible for the development of hypoalbuminemia as an origin for peripheral edema (see **Table 5**).

REFERENCES

1. Bradley EL III, Isaacs JT, Mazo JD, et al. Pathophysiology and significance of malabsorption after Roux-en-Y reconstruction. Surgery 1977;81:684–91.
2. Ervin RB. Prevalence of metabolic syndrome among adults 20 years of age and over, by sex, age, race, and ethnicity, and body mass index: United States, 2003–2006. Natl Health Stat Report 2009;13:1–7.
3. Batsis JA, Romero-Corral A, Collazo-Clavell ML, et al. Effect of bariatric surgery on the metabolic syndrome: a population-based, long-term controlled study. Mayo Clin Proc 2008;83(8):897–907.
4. Roddy DR, Koch TR, Reilly WM, et al. Identification and distribution of peptide YY in the human, canine, and murine gastrointestinal tracts: species-related antibody recognition differences. Regul Pept 1987;18:201–12.
5. Baggio LL, Drucker DJ. Biology of incretins: GLP-1 and GIP. Gastroenterology 2007;132:2131–57.
6. Mingrone G. Role of the incretin system in the remission of type 2 diabetes following bariatric surgery. Nutr Metab Cardiovasc Dis 2008;18(8):574–9.
7. Peterli R, Wolnerhanssen B, Peters T, et al. Improvement in glucose metabolism after bariatric surgery: comparison of laparoscopic Roux-en-Y gastric bypass and laparoscopic sleeve gastrectomy: a prospective randomized trial. Ann Surg 2009;250(2):234–41.
8. Korner J, Bessler M, Inabnet W, et al. Exaggerated glucagons-like peptide-1 and blunted glucose-dependent insulinotrophic peptide secretion are associated with

Roux-en-Y gastric bypass but not adjustable gastric banding. Surg Obes Relat Dis 2007;3(6):597–601.

9. Korner J, Inabnet W, Febres G, et al. Prospective study of gut hormone and metabolic changes after adjustable gastric banding and Roux-en-Y gastric bypass. Int J Obes (Lond) 2009;33(7):786–95.

10. Buchwald H, Estok R, Fahrbach K, et al. Weight and type 2 diabetes after bariatric surgery: systematic review and meta-analysis. Am J Med 2009;122(3):248–56.

11. Lin E, Davis SS, Srinivasan J, et al. Dual mechanisms for type-2 diabetes resolution after Roux-en-Y gastric bypass. Am Surg 2009;75:498–502.

12. Kadera BE, Lum K, Grant J, et al. Remission of type 2 diabetes after Roux-en-Y gastric bypass is associated with greater weight loss. Surg Obes Relat Dis 2009; 5(3):305–9.

13. Dixon JB, O'Brien PE, Playfair J, et al. Adjustable gastric banding and conventional therapy for type 2 diabetes: a randomized controlled trial. JAMA 2008; 299(3):316–23.

14. Kim SH, Liu TC, Abbasi F, et al. Plasma glucose and insulin regulation is abnormal following gastric bypass surgery with or without neuroglycopenia. Obes Surg 2009;19(11):1550–6.

15. Spanakis E, Gragnoli C. Successful medical management of status post-Roux-en-Y-gastric-bypass hyperinsulinemic hypoglycemia. Obes Surg 2009;19(9):1333–4.

16. Moreira RO, Moreira RB, Machado NA, et al. Post-prandial hypoglycemia after bariatric surgery: pharmacological treatment with verapamil and acarbose. Obes Surg 2008;18(12):1618–21.

17. Gehring N, Imoberdorf R, Wegmann M, et al. Serum albumin—a qualified parameter to determine the nutritional status? Swiss Med Wkly 2006;136:664–9.

18. Don BR, Kaysen G. Serum albumin: relationship to inflammation and nutrition. Semin Dial 2004;17:432–7.

19. Machado JD, Campos CS, Lopes Dah Silva C, et al. Intestinal bacterial overgrowth after Roux-en-Y gastric bypass. Obes Surg 2008;18(1):139–43.

20. Lewandowski H, Breen TL, Huang EY. Kwashiorkor and an acrodermatitis enteropathica-like eruption after a distal gastric bypass surgical procedure. Endocr Pract 2007;13(3):277–82.

21. Aasheim ET, Bjorkman S, Sevik TT, et al. Vitamin status after bariatric surgery: a randomized study of gastric bypass and duodenal switch. Am J Clin Nutr 2009;90(1):15–22.

22. Toh SY, Zarshenas N, Jorgensen J, et al. Prevalence of nutrient deficiencies in bariatric patients. Nutrition 2009;25(11–12):1150–6.

23. Johnson JM, Maher JW, Samuel I, et al. Effects of gastric bypass procedures on bone mineral density, calcium, parathyroid hormone, and vitamin D. J Gastrointest Surg 2005;9:1106–11.

24. Johnson JM, Maher JW, DeMaria EJ, et al. The long-term effects of gastric bypass on Vitamin D metabolism. Ann Surg 2006;243(5):701–5.

25. Dawson-Hughes B, Heaney RP, Holick MF, et al. Estimates of optimal vitamin D status. Osteoporos Int 2005;16(7):713–6.

26. Bendich A, Machlin LJ. Safety of oral intake of vitamin E. Am J Clin Nutr 1988;48:612–9.

27. Shearer MJ, McBurney A, Barkhan P. Studies on the absorption and metabolism of phylloquine (vitamin K) in man. Vitam Horm 1974;32:513–4.

28. Lakhani SV, Shah HN, Alexander K, et al. Small intestinal bacterial overgrowth and thiamine deficiency after Roux-en-Y gastric bypass surgery in obese patients. Nutr Res 2008;28(5):293–8.

29. Herve C, Beyne P, Letteron P, et al. Comparison of erythrocyte transketolase activity with thiamine and thiamine phosphate ester levels in chronic alcoholic patients. Clin Chim Acta 1995;234(1–2):91–100.

30. Thomson AD, Marshall EJ. The treatment of patients at risk of developing Wernicke's encephalopathy in the community. Alcohol Alcohol 2006;41:159–67.

31. Koch TR, Yuan L-X, Fink JG, et al. Induction of enlarged intestinal lymphoid aggregates during acute glutathione depletion in a murine model. Dig Dis Sci 2000;45(11):2115–21.

32. German AJ, Day MJ, Ruaux CG, et al. Comparison of direct and indirect tests for small intestinal bacterial overgrowth and antibiotic-responsive diarrhea in dogs. J Vet Intern Med 2003;17(1):33–43.

33. Rutgers HC, Batt RM, Elwood CM, et al. Small intestinal bacterial overgrowth in dogs with chronic intestinal disease. J Am Vet Med Assoc 1995;206(2):187–93.

34. Vargas-Ruiz AG, Hernández-Rivera G, Herrera MF. Prevalence of iron, folate, and vitamin B12 deficiency anemia after laparoscopic Roux-en-Y gastric bypass. Obes Surg 2008;18(3):288–93.

35. Herrmann W, Obeid R. Causes and early diagnosis of vitamin B12 deficiency. Dtsch Arztebl Int 2008;105(40):680–5.

36. Powell SR. The antioxidant properties of zinc. J Nutr 2000;130:1447S–54S.

37. DiSilvestro RA. Zinc in relation to diabetes and oxidative stress. J Nutr 2000;130:1509S–11S.

38. Oury TD, Day BJ, Crapo JD. Extracellular superdioxide dismutase: a regulator of nitric oxide availability. Lab Invest 1996;75:617–36.

39. Yu HH, Shan YS, Lin PW. Zinc deficiency with acrodermatitis enteropathica-like eruption after pancreaticoduodenectomy. J Formos Med Assoc 2007;106:864–8.

40. Johnson VJ, Tsunoda M, Sharma RP. Increased production of proinflammatory cytokines by murine macrophages following oral exposure to sodium selenite but not to seleno-L-methionine. Arch Environ Contam Toxicol 2000;39:243–50.

41. Hill GM, Link JE. Transporters in the absorption and utilization of zinc and copper. J Anim Sci 2009;87:E85–9.

42. Kumar N, Ahlskog JE, Gross JB Jr. Acquired hypocupremia after gastric surgery. Clin Gastroenterol Hepatol 2004;2:1074–9.

43. Kumar N. Copper deficiency myelopathy (human swayback). Mayo Clin Proc 2006;81:1371–84.

44. Marinella MA. Anemia following Roux-en-Y surgery for morbid obesity: a review. South Med J 2008;101:1024–31.

45. Von Drygalski A, Andris DA. Anemia after bariatric surgery: more than just iron deficiency. Nutr Clin Pract 2009;24:217–26.

46. Koffman BM, Greenfield LJ, Ali II, et al. Neurologic complications after surgery for obesity. Muscle Nerve 2006;33:166–76.

The Surgical Treatment of Metabolic Disease and Morbid Obesity

Mark A. Fontana, MD[a,b,*], Stephen D. Wohlgemuth, MD[a,b]

KEYWORDS

• Bariatric • Surgery • Bypass • Sleeve • Treatment

The disease of obesity has continued to increase in the United States. Obesity is defined as a body mass index (BMI) greater than 30 kg/m^2. In 1991, the National Institute of Health Consensus Panel on Gastric Surgery for Severe Obesity defined the population who would most likely benefit from bariatric surgery. These same criteria continue to be used today to determine which patients should undergo metabolic and weight loss surgery. These recommendations include patients who have a BMI greater than 35 kg/m^2 with significant comorbid conditions such as diabetes, hypertension, or obstructive sleep apnea; and patients who have a BMI greater than 40 kg/m^2 with or without any significant comorbid conditions because they have a significant increased risk for developing these conditions.

Over the past 20 years the rate of obesity has shown a dramatic increase. The most recent statistics show that 32 states now have obesity rates greater than 25% of the adult population. Six states have obesity rates greater than 30% of the adult population and only one state, Colorado, has an obesity rate less than 20%. This means that 72 million American adults have a body mass index (BMI) of 30 kg/m^2 or greater. A closer evaluation of the statistics shows that a significant BMI shift has occurred so that the entire adult population is heavier. More worrisome is that the heaviest people have become much heavier over the past 20 years. Furthermore, disparities clearly exist among racial and ethnic populations, with a disproportionately high number of non-Hispanic black and Mexican American women in the morbid obesity range.[1]

No significant improvements have occurred in the dietary approach to long-term weight loss over the past few years. Several dietary medications are still available; however, the success rate of dieting with behavioral changes alone and in combination with medications continues to be in the single digits.

Bariatric surgery has gained widespread acceptance. Evidence continues to show that it is the only treatment currently available with significant cure rates for diseases

^{a} Sentara Metabolic and Weight Loss Surgery Center, 600 Gresham Drive, Suite 8630, Norfolk, VA 23507, USA
^{b} Eastern Virginia Medical School, Norfolk, VA, USA
* Corresponding author.
E-mail address: mafontan@sentara.com (M.A. Fontana).

Gastroenterol Clin N Am 39 (2010) 125–133
doi:10.1016/j.gtc.2009.12.010
0889-8553/10/$ – see front matter © 2010 Elsevier Inc. All rights reserved.

such as diabetes, hypertension, and heart failure, and myriad other comorbid conditions associated with obesity. Increasing evidence shows significant risk reduction for many cancers associated with obesity within 1 year of the significant weight loss associated with metabolic surgery.[2]

Although bariatric surgery has been performed for more than 40 years, in 1995 Pories and colleagues[3] showed that the procedure provided durable weight loss of more than 100 pounds, significant improvement in comorbidities, including diabetes, and a decrease in overall mortality among 608 patients who underwent gastric bypass over 14 years.[3] Since that seminal report, surgery began to gain more acceptance as a viable treatment option.

In 1994, Clark and Wittgrove showed that gastric bypass could be performed safely laparoscopically and now most gastric bypasses and nearly all gastric banding procedures are performed using this technique. Finally, the nationwide acceptance of centers of excellence credentialed by the American College of Surgeons and the Surgical Review Corporation, where high volumes of surgery are performed by experienced surgeons, has proven that surgical risk and complications can be kept to an acceptably minimal level.

In a recent study, the LABS consortium[4] reviewed 30-day outcomes from 10 centers for 4610 surgical procedures: 3412 gastric bypass and 1198 laparoscopic adjustable gastric bandings. The combined 30-day mortality was 0.3%, with a major complication rate of only 4.3%.

Lastly, although bariatric surgery has a higher risk than the nonoperative treatments of obesity, the definition of success is more stringently applied. For the nonoperative treatment of obesity, a 10% excess body weight loss maintained for 1 year is considered successful; this would be equal to a 220-pound patient, whose ideal weight is 120 pounds, losing 10 pounds and maintaining that weight loss for 1 year. The likelihood of this success is approximately 5%, with a 95% rate of failure. The definition of success for bariatric surgery is a loss of at least 50% of the excess body weight. Pooled data show a 54% to 67% excess body weight loss, depending on the type of surgery, that is maintained over a 10-year period with no evidence of loss of effect.[5]

This article reviews the weight loss surgery options, beginning with the common operations performed currently, and then briefly discussing operations that are no longer performed.

OPERATIONS COMMONLY PERFORMED CURRENTLY
Roux-en-Y Gastric Bypass

Roux-en-Y gastric bypass is the most commonly performed bariatric operation in the United States (**Fig. 1**). It is considered the gold standard operation to which all other operations are compared. It can be performed in a laparoscopic or the traditional open technique. This procedure considered restrictive and malabsorptive. The restrictive component to this operation entails creating a 20- to 30-mL gastric pouch just below the gastroesophageal junction. This pouch is either partitioned from the lower portion of the stomach or, more commonly, completely divided away from the lower, remnant stomach. The jejunum is then divided 30 to 50 cm distal to the ligament of Treitz, and the distal side of this division brought into the upper abdomen and anastomosed to the gastric pouch. This anastomosis can be performed with staplers or by simple sewing techniques. The proximal jejunal limb, which carries gastric secretions and biliopancreatic secretions, is then anastomosed back to the jejunum 75 to 150 cm from the gastrojejunal anastomosis. This technique provides the

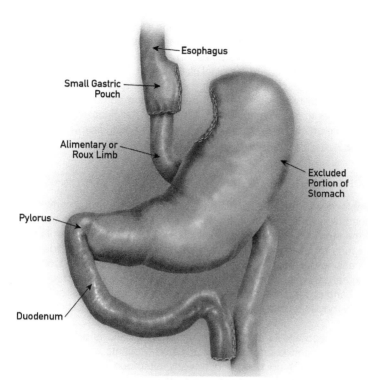

Esophagus

Small Gastric Pouch

Alimentary or Roux Limb

Excluded Portion of Stomach

Pylorus

Duodenum

Fig. 1. Roux-en-Y gastric bypass. (*Courtesy of* Ethicon Endo-Surgery, Inc; with permission.)

malabsorptive component of the operation by preventing the mixing of food and digestive enzymes as food or drink traverses the Roux limb.

Because the laparoscopic approach has become the most common method of gastric bypass and completely divides the gastric pouch away from the distal, remnant stomach, the complication of staple-line dehiscence or gastro–gastric fistula will likely become far less common. The complete separation of the distal remnant stomach makes it much more difficult to access using an endoscopic technique. In addition, benefits of the laparoscopic approach include shorter hospitalization, decreased pain, and significant reduction in the rate of abdominal wall hernia.

Results and Outcomes

Roux-en-Y gastric bypass is a very effective operation, and the authors routinely see 50% excess body weight loss in the first 6 months after surgery. An approximately 75% excess body weight loss is common over the first 18 months, with an approximately 10% weight regain by the fourth or fifth year postoperatively.

As for comorbidity resolution, in a meta-analysis involving 136 studies with 22,000 patients, Buchwald and colleagues[6] showed improvement in fasting blood glucose and hemoglobin A1C in 83% of patients, improvement of hyperlipidemia in 87% of patients, resolution of hypertension in 67.5% patients, and resolution or improvement of sleep apnea in 94% of patients.

Although the overall complication rate has been reported to be as high as 24%, it involves a significant portion of minor complications, such as early postoperative dehydration and nausea.[7] The rate of major complications, such as deep vein thrombosis, pulmonary embolism, and bleeding requiring a transfusion or readmission to the hospital, is approximately 9%. The mortality rate for gastric bypass has been reported to be between 0.5% and 2% in all studies.[7] The most common long-term complications include internal hernias and marginal ulceration at the gastrojejunal anastamosis. Postoperative nutritional deficiencies depend on several factors, such preoperative nutritional status, ability to modify eating behavior, and compliance with prescribed vitamin and mineral supplementation.[8] Nutritional deficiencies are discussed in more detail in the article by Koch and colleagues appearing elsewhere in this issue.

LAPAROSCOPIC ADJUSTABLE GASTRIC BANDING

The adjustable gastric band was first developed by Kuzmak[9] in the early 1980s. It was a later refined to include a saline-filled bladder within a band that encircles the upper portion of the stomach in a belt-like fashion. The saline-filled bladder is attached to tubing that runs to a reservoir in the subcutaneous tissue. The bladder is adjusted through accessing the reservoir (**Fig. 2**). The band that encircles the stomach creates a small proximal gastric pouch, which can hold 2 to 3 ounces of solid food. The outflow through the band is adjusted through adding saline through the subcutaneous reservoir. The band therefore limits intake by causing a rapid feeling of satiety with relatively small meals.

A decrease in appetite is also commonly reported, and is noticed by almost all patients when the band is appropriately adjusted. Patients who have well-adjusted bands frequently report no hunger until early afternoon or even later. They also routinely eat only two meals per day that are relatively small volume in size.

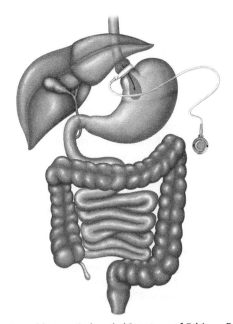

Fig. 2. Laparoscopic adjustable gastric band. (*Courtesy of* Ethicon Endo-Surgery, Inc; with permission.)

Result and Outcomes

The laparoscopic adjustable gastric band has the lowest complication rate of all bariatric operations, with a 12% rate of late complications, such as gastric prolapse, erosion, or infection; a 5% 30-day postoperative morbidity rate; and a 0.05% mortality rate.[10]

The most common long-term complication after laparoscopic adjustable gastric banding is gastric prolapse/band slippage, with band erosion or other infectious complications seen more rarely. Gastric prolapse consists of herniation of the stomach up through the band, resulting in a larger gastric pouch, malpositioning of the band, and eventual partial or complete occlusion of the band. Band erosion into the gastric lumen is a rare complication.

Patients who have laparoscopic adjustable gastric banding can expect to lose more than 50% of their extra body weight over 3 years. Longer-term studies show that weight loss with laparoscopic adjustable band is durable, with an 83% success rate for maintaining 50% loss of extra body weight for at least 5 years or more.[11]

Comorbidity resolution is slightly lower with laparoscopic banding than with gastric bypass. Individual studies show up to 80% resolution or significant improvement of diabetes after laparoscopic adjustable gastric band. However, the meta-analysis by Buchwald and colleagues[6] showed resolution or significant improvement of diabetes in 47.9% of patients compared with 83.7% of patients who underwent gastric bypass. O'Brien and colleagues[12] found that patients experienced a 74% improvement or resolution of dyslipidemia, 94% resolution of obstructive sleep apnea, 55% resolution of hypertension, and 76% resolution of gastroesophageal reflux disease.

BILIOPANCREATIC DIVERSION AND BILIOPANCREATIC DIVERSION WITH DUODENAL SWITCH

The biliopancreatic diversion (BPD) was first described by Scopinaro and colleagues[13] in 1979 and remains one of the most effective weight loss operations. The procedure consists of a subtotal gastrectomy with creation of an approximately 200 to 500 mL gastric pouch. Intestinal continuity is restored through formation of a Roux-en-Y gastro-ileostomy of approximately 200 cm with a common channel of approximately 50 cm. A small amount of restriction is created by the decreased gastric reservoir and a significant amount of malabsorption that is primarily selective for fat and starch. Although excellent weight loss has been achieved, significant complications have occurred, including iron deficiency anemia, bone demineralization secondary to decreased calcium absorption, and stomal ulceration. Additionally, an increased incidence of protein malnutrition has been seen.

In 1988, Hess and colleagues[14] and Marceau and colleagues[15] simultaneously described a new procedure combining features of the original BPD and an earlier operation called the duodenal switch (DS), which had been introduced by DeMeester[16] in 1987. The restrictive portion of the procedure involves the creation of a vertical sleeve gastrectomy of approximately 100 to 150 mL (**Fig. 3**). The duodenum is then transected in the first portion and a duodenal ileostomy created, with a resultant 150-cm alimentary limb and a common channel of 100 cm. The combination of the sleeve gastrectomy and the length of the common channel have significantly decreased many of the complications seen with the original BPD, such as hyperproteinemia, anastamotic ulcers, hypocalcemia, and anemia.

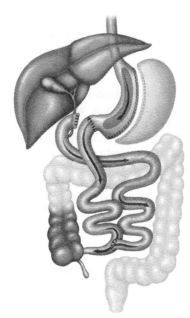

Fig. 3. Biliopancreatic diversion with duodenal switch. (*Courtesy of* Ethicon Endo-Surgery, Inc; with permission.)

Results and Outcomes

Weight loss associated with BPD and BPD/DS has been greater than with any other currently performed bariatric procedure. Excess weight loss of 70% to 80% has been achieved long-term, associated with very acceptable nutritional complications.[15] BPD and BPD/DS have become the preferred procedures in many bariatric centers for treating patients who have a BMI greater than 50 kg/m^2. Excellent resolution of comorbidities has been associated with this weight loss, with a 98% cure rate for type 2 diabetes.[15]

The complications associated with these procedures are similar to those found with a Roux-en-Y gastric bypass, such as anastamotic leaks, bleeding, and bowel obstruction. Careful attention to long-term mineral and vitamin supplementation is essential to prevent nutritional complications. Because the BPD and BPD/DS more technically demanding than a bypass or band, and are frequently performed on super-morbidly obese patients, mortality rates have been higher than those reported with bypass or banding.[15]

SLEEVE GASTRECTOMY

The sleeve gastrectomy or vertical gastrectomy involves the creation of a long tubular gastric conduit based on the lesser curve of the stomach (**Fig. 4**). Most of the fundus and body of the stomach are resected with preservation of the gastric antrum. The total volume of the resultant gastric sleeve is approximately 100 to 150 mL. Initial reports of the sleeve gastrectomy primarily involved patients at extremely high risk for conventional bariatric surgery.[17] Experts believed that a laparoscopic sleeve gastrectomy would allow 100-pound weight loss in 6 to 9 months, allowing for a second bariatric surgery such as a gastric bypass or BPD/DS.

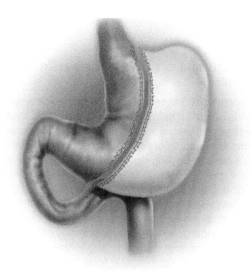

Fig. 4. Sleeve gastrectomy. (*Courtesy of* Ethicon Endo-Surgery, Inc; with permission.)

This approach has been shown to be successful in numerous series. In a series of high-risk patients who had an average BMI of 65.3 kg/m^2, Cottam and colleagues[18] reported that approximately 1 year after a laparoscopic sleeve gastrectomy, the mean BMI had decreased to 49 kg/m^2, with a significant decrease in comorbidities. Most of these patients went on to a second-stage gastric bypass, which was performed with a very acceptable rate of complications and no mortality.

Since 2006, an increasing body of literature has supported the use of a sleeve gastrectomy as a primary standalone bariatric procedure.[19] The reasons for this include its relative ease compared with a bypass or DS, lack of an anastomosis, avoidance of a foreign body, and absence of need for postoperative adjustments.

Results and Outcomes

Brethauer and colleagues[20] recently published a systematic review of sleeve gastrectomy as both a part of a staged and as a primary operation. They reviewed 36 studies involving 2570 patients. Patients who underwent a sleeve gastrectomy as the first stage of a staged procedure had an average preoperative BMI of 60 kg/m^2 and excess weight loss of 47%. This high-risk group had complication rates of 1.2% for leakS, 1.6% for bleeding, 0.9% for stricture, and 0.24% for mortality. When a sleeve gastrectomy was performed as a primary procedure, the mean BMI was 46.6 kg/m^2 and the mean percent excess weight loss was 60% with a mean follow-up of 32 months. Complication rates were 2.7% leaks, 1.0% bleeding, and 0.5% strictures. The mortality rate was 0.17%. Although limited long-term data are available, some studies do have 3- and 5-year data that show good durability.

The sleeve gastrectomy seems to be a very viable standalone operation, with excellent weight loss and comorbidity resolution comparable to currently accepted bariatric procedures. The current feeling is that the sleeve gastrectomy is safer than a bypass but not as safe as a band, and is associated with more weight loss than a band but not as much as a bypass. It could become the preferred procedure for patients concerned about the long-term nutritional consequences of the malabsorptive procedures, or those uncomfortable with the risks associated with an implanted foreign body, such as patients who undergo transplantation who are in need of long-term immunosuppression.

LESS COMMON AND HISTORICAL OPERATIONS FOR WEIGHT LOSS
Vertical Banded Gastroplasty

Vertical banded gastroplasty (VBG) was the first accepted surgical weight loss procedure. It was the most common operation before the Roux-en-Y gastric bypass, and has largely been replaced by the laparoscopic adjustable gastric band. VBG created a 30- to 50-mL gastric pouch along the lesser curve of the stomach from the angle of Hiss to a circular opening created with a circular stapling device. A 5-cm long piece of Marlex mesh was then placed around the gastric pouch to create a permanently limited outflow tract to the gastric antrum. Although this operation showed excellent 1-year results, after 3 to 5 years only 40% of patients were able to maintain a 50% excess body weight loss, and longer-term follow-up showed a further reduction of effectiveness.[21]

Many patient have still undergone VBG. Complications commonly reported include stomal stenosis frequently requiring dilatation, staple-line disruption with a complete loss of the restrictive nature of the surgery, food bolus obstructions, and severe esophagitis.

Conversion of VBG to Roux-en-Y gastric bypass is one of the more commonly performed revision bariatric surgeries.

Jejunoileal Bypass

Jejunoileal bypass, first described in the 1960s, was a malabsorptive procedure in which a 35-cm biliopancreatic limb of proximal jejunum was anastomosed to the terminal ileum 10 cm from the ileocecal valve. Although this procedure had excellent weight loss results, the long-term complications, including intractable diarrhea, electrolyte imbalances, calcium oxalate kidney stones, hypoalbuminemia, and liver failure, caused it to be abandoned by the end of the 1980s. Nearly 25,000 jejunoileal bypasses were performed, and most have been converted to gastric bypass or normal anatomy because of these complications.

SUMMARY

There has never been a time when so many viable alternatives for metabolic and weight loss surgery were available. Currently four well-accepted procedures are performed: the Roux-en-Y gastric bypass, laparoscopic adjustable band, sleeve gastrectomy, and biliopancreatic diversion. Evidence shows that each of these procedures is associated with excellent long-term weight loss compared with every nonsurgical alternative, and each has a reasonably low complication profile. The emphasis now is on matching the appropriate patient with the appropriate surgery. These surgical procedures have very few strict contraindications. The authors believe that well-educated patients and thoughtful physicians can choose the appropriate surgery.

Clearly, pitfalls exist that can cause any of these surgical procedures to fail. The importance of patient compliance with postsurgical diet and exercise programs cannot be underestimated. Patients must understand that their bariatric surgery is a tool that, when used correctly, can lead to long-term weight loss, comorbidity resolution, and improvement in quality and quantity of life. Appropriate selection of patients is critical for bariatric surgery, which involves a comprehensive preoperative assessment to evaluate eating or behavioral disorders, metabolic disease, and associated comorbidities. Patients must also understand that they will need lifelong ongoing regular follow-up with their surgeon.

REFERENCES

1. Ogden C, Carrol M, McDowell M, et al. Obesity among adults in the United States—no statistically significant change since 2003-2004. NCHS Data Brief 2007;1:1–5.
2. Adams TD, Gress RE, Smith SC, et al. Long-term mortality after gastric bypass surgery. N Engl J Med 2007;357:753–61.
3. Pories WJ, Swanson MS, MacDonald KG, et al. Who would have thought it? An operation proves to be the most effective therapy for adult-onset diabetes mellitus. Ann Surg 1995;222:339–52.
4. Longitudinal Assessment of Bariatric Surgery (LABS) consortium. Perioperative safety in the longitudinal assessment of bariatric surgery. N Engl J Med 2009; 361:445–54.
5. O'Brien PE, McPhail T, Chaston TB, et al. Systemic review of medium-term weight loss after bariatric operations. Obes Surg 2006;16:1032–40.
6. Buchwald H, Avidor Y, Braunwald E, et al. Bariatric surgery: a systematic review and meta-analysis. JAMA 2004;292:1724–37.
7. Parikh M, Ren CJ, Laker S. Objective comparison of complications resulting from laparoscopic bariatric procedures. J Am Coll Surg 2006;202:252–61.
8. Tucker O, Szomstein S, Rosenthal S. Nutritional consequences of weight-loss surgery. Med Clin North Am 2007;91:499–514.
9. Kuzmak LI. A review of seven years' experience with silicone gastric banding. Obes Surg 1991;1:403–8.
10. Fielding GA, Ren CJ. Laparoscopic adjustable gastric band. Surg Clin North Am 2005;85:129–40.
11. O'Brien PE, Mcphail T. Systematic review of medium-term weight loss after bariatric operations. Obes Surg 2006;16:1032–40.
12. O'Brien PE, Dixon JB, Smith A. The laparoscopic adjustable gastric band: a prospective study of medium term effects on weight, health and quality of life. Obes Surg 2002;12:652–60.
13. Scopinaro N, Gianetta E, Civalleri D, et al. Bilio-pancreatic by-pass for obesity. (I and II). Br J Surg 1979;66:616–20.
14. Hess DS, Hess DW. Biliopancreatic diversion with a duodenal switch. Obes Surg 1998;8:267–82.
15. Marceau P, Hould FS, Simard S, et al. Biliopancreatic diversion with duodenal switch. World J Surg 1998;22:947–54.
16. DeMeester TR, Fuchs KH, Ball CS, et al. Experimental and clinical results with proximal end-to-end duodenojejunostomy for pathologic duodenogastric reflux. Ann Surg 1987;206:414–26.
17. Regan JP, Inabnet WB, Gagner M, et al. Early experience with two-stage laparoscopic Roux-en-Y gastric bypass as an alternative in the super-super obese patient. Obes Surg 2003;13:861–4.
18. Cottam D, Queshi FG, Mattar SG, et al. Laparoscopic sleeve gastrectomy as an initial weight-loss procedure for high-risk patients with morbid obesity. Surg Endosc 2006;20:859–63.
19. Lee CM, Cirangle PT, Jossart GH. Vertical gastrectomy for morbid obesity in 216 patients: report of two-year results. Surg Endosc 2007;21:1810–6.
20. Brethauer SA, Hammel JP, Schauer PR. Systematic review of sleeve gastrectomy as staging and primary bariatric procedure. Surg Obes Relat Dis 2009;5:469–75.
21. Maclean LD. Late results of vertical banded gastroplasty for morbid and super obesity. Surgery 1990;107:20–7.

Short- and Long-Term Surgical Follow-Up of the Postbariatric Surgery Patient

Paul Frank, Peter F. Crookes, MD*

KEYWORDS

- Malnutrition • Vitamin deficiency • Reflux
- Outcomes • Bariatric • Follow-up

Historically, it was customary for patients requiring surgery to be referred to a surgeon by an internist. The surgeon performed the procedure requested by the referring physician, and surgical follow-up was limited to ensuring that the patient had healed from the effects of the surgery and that perioperative complications were adequately managed. The long-term management of the underlying disease remained the responsibility of the internist. A major change in emphasis has occurred as more and more benign diseases requiring lifelong attention are managed by surgical therapy. The process began with the long-term studies on the outcome of surgery for peptic ulcer disease originating in centers such as Leeds, England, in the middle of the twentieth century. During the same time period Ronald Belsey in Bristol, England, inculcated the same concept in generations of thoracic surgeons treating hiatal hernia and reflux disease. It is no accident that these principles began to be learned shortly after the introduction of the British National Health Service in 1948. The radically different structure of health care in the United States is not as amenable to long-term follow-up of patients because there is no central way of collecting the data, and repetitive visits for many years are viewed as unnecessary and costly unless driven by specific symptoms or risk factors. Nevertheless, in conditions in which surgical therapy induces permanent alteration in physiology, there is increasing recognition that the surgeon is in a good position to understand the pathophysiology of the condition and the physiologic consequences of the operative procedure and that the surgeon is the ideal person to provide long-term follow-up. There is no area of medical practice where this is truer than for bariatric surgery. The major societies promoting the science and practice of bariatric surgery, notably the American Society for Metabolic and Bariatric Surgery (ASMBS), have been leaders in the surgical community in creating

Department of Surgery, Keck School of Medicine, University of Southern California, 1510 San Pablo Street, Suite 514, Los Angeles, CA 90033, USA
* Corresponding author.
E-mail address: pcrookes@surgery.usc.edu

Gastroenterol Clin N Am 39 (2010) 135–146
doi:10.1016/j.gtc.2009.12.011
0889-8553/10/$ – see front matter © 2010 Elsevier Inc. All rights reserved.

gastro.theclinics.com

a culture where long-term structured follow-up of patients after bariatric surgery is the responsibility of the operating surgeon. This ideal goal is still a work in progress. It is inevitable that many patients undergoing bariatric surgery will eventually be cared for by other physicians, and knowledge of the anatomy and physiology of bariatric procedures is essential for modern internists. Good communication links with bariatric surgeons also facilitates the care of this challenging population of patients.

DEFINITIONS

This review concentrates on the 3 major bariatric procedures commonly performed in this country for severe obesity and its comorbidities. The most commonly performed operation is the Roux-en-Y gastric bypass (RYGB), which accounts for about 65% of contemporary procedures, and laparoscopic adjustable gastric banding (LAGB) accounts for about 25%. The remaining 10% include procedures such as the duodenal switch (DS) or its precursor biliopancreatic diversion (BPD) and, more recently, the sleeve gastrectomy.[1] The details of these procedures are described elsewhere in this issue and therefore not be repeated here. However, primary care providers should have a broad understanding of the principles of these different procedures because each produces a different spectrum of complications and side effects.

Follow-up after surgery can be conveniently grouped into 3 phases, namely short term (up to 3 months from surgery), medium term (3–24 months), and longer term (>2–5 years). These definitions are to some extent arbitrary, but the principles are broadly agreed upon.

SHORT-TERM FOLLOW-UP

Short-term follow-up is largely aimed at ensuring that the patient heals without any perioperative complications. This is so fundamental that all postoperative visits within 90 days of any surgical procedure are regarded by third party payers as being within the global period covered by the surgeon's fee. During this period, the focus of the visits is to monitor the healing of incisions and to ensure that there are no leaks and that function in the new stomach reconstruction is adequate to avoid critical problems such as dehydration and vitamin deficiency. Patients are typically scheduled for routine postoperative visits 2 and 6 weeks after discharge from hospital.

Serious perioperative complications are managed initially as inpatients by the surgeon. The most serious complications are leaks from the anastomosis or other suture lines (about 1%–2% in contemporary series) and pulmonary embolism (less than 1%).[2] Patients recovering from such complications are followed up much more closely and may require prolonged courses of intravenous (IV) antibiotics and possibly total parenteral nutrition and follow-up computed tomography (CT)-guided drain placement. Taking care of drainage tubes and managing open wounds then dominate the early postoperative visits. Pain management, physical therapy, and nutritional supervision also require much more attention in such patients.

In the absence of such serious complications, the problems arising during the first 3 months after surgery typically are classified into 3 categories:

Incisional Problems

The incidence of surgical site infection (SSI) may be 10% or even higher after open bariatric surgery [3] Risk factors include high body mass index (BMI), poorly controlled diabetes, smoking, and the duration (and indirectly, the difficulty) of the procedure. Timely administration of appropriate antibiotics (less than 60 minutes before making the skin incision and discontinuance within 24 hours of surgery) has reduced the incidence to some extent. Tight control of blood sugar and avoidance of hypothermia intraoperatively and administration of a high fraction of inspired oxygen (F$_{IO_2}$) in the recovery ward immediately after surgery may also help reduce the risk of SSI, but the value of these measures remains controversial. SSI typically develops 5 to 10 days after surgery and is rarely obvious before the patient goes home, typically on postoperative day 3 to 5. Patients often present a few days after discharge with redness or induration in part of the incision, associated with systemic signs of fever, tachycardia, and worsening gastrointestinal (GI) function. In contrast, laparoscopic incisions are rarely complicated by infection. However, when a circular stapler is used to fashion the gastrojejunal (GJ) anastomosis, the surgeon must enlarge one of the trocar sites to permit introduction of the stapling cartridge, and after the cartridge is fired, it may be difficult to avoid contaminating the wound edge as it is removed from the abdomen. Infection of that particular port site occasionally occurs in that situation.

Early GI Dysfunction

The narrow gastric pouch after RYGB or sleeve gastrectomy is restrictive at the beginning, and patients can usually tolerate only clear liquids in small quantities at first. Patients are usually given written instructions to guide the gradual increase in the quantity and range of foods they can tolerate. Patients who do not receive or who do not understand such instruction have a high incidence of vomiting postoperatively. Many patients will experience a few episodes of vomiting if they relax the vigilance with which they increase their dietary intake, and some vomiting is probably inevitable as they learn how to cope with a sensation of fullness, which is a novel experience for most bariatric patients. However, in well-instructed and supported patients, it should be rare. Rather than berate the patient for failure of compliance, or attribute vomiting to persistence of a psychological compulsion to eat large quantities quickly, the physician should consider organic causes, namely a stricture. Some degree of stricturing of the GJ anastomosis is common, and usually resolves with time (less than 3 months) and can be managed by going back to softer or liquid foods. A more severe stricture may be because of an ulcer at the anastomosis, and the physician should inquire about consumption of nonsteroidal antiinflammatory drugs (NSAIDs) or large pills or resumption of smoking. Endoscopy typically reveals an ulcer with visible suture material or staples (**Fig. 1**). Such strictures are easy to dilate, and 1 or 2 dilations generally are sufficient.

The effects of persistent vomiting may be serious, and vomiting may lead to dehydration and renal impairment. This is usually quickly reversible. A rare but much more serious result of persistent vomiting is Wernicke encephalopathy, which is a consequence of thiamine deficiency. It is characterized by changes in mental status (confusion, short-term memory loss), ataxia, and eye movement signs such as nystagmus and ophthalmoplegia. A recent review described 104 cases, with the majority presenting between 1 and 3 months postoperatively.[4] Confirmation by measuring thiamine levels is not routinely done because blood levels are not always subnormal and are rarely available in time to help the diagnosis. Therefore, this diagnosis should be considered in any patient after recent bariatric surgery who presents with changes in mental status, and it should be remembered that administration of dextrose can worsen the situation. Thus immediate administration of thiamine (100 mg IV or intramuscular) is advisable in any patient reporting frequent vomiting in the first few months after bariatric surgery.

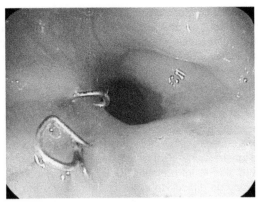

Fig. 1. Endoscopic appearance of an anastomotic stricture with visible staples but without ulceration.

Bile vomiting early after bypass surgery is almost unheard of unless there is a major problem with the reconstruction, such as a mechanical obstruction just beyond the enteroenterostomy or even the "Roux-en-O" pattern, where the biliopancreatic limb was mistaken for the Roux limb and connected to the stomach. Bile vomiting is highly likely to mandate a reoperation, and if the original surgeon is reluctant to undertake it, the internist should refer the patient to a major referral center.[5]

Lower GI tract dysfunction may result in diarrhea, and if the diarrhea is persistent, it is important to check for *Clostridium difficile* toxin. Diarrhea is common after malabsorptive operations, such as the DS, whereas constipation is common after gastric bypass. These complications tend to resolve with time as dietary intake becomes more varied. Simple over-the-counter remedies are occasionally needed in this situation.

Management of Coexisting Medical Problems

Many patients are already on treatment for comorbid problems such as hypertension, diabetes, hyperlipidemia, depression, and other conditions unrelated to obesity. There is often confusion about how these conditions should be managed, because surgeons may not be comfortable adjusting the doses of antihypertensives or hypoglycemic agents and the internist may not be aware of the physical restrictions imposed by different kinds of reconstruction.

In general, swallowing large pills within the first 6 weeks of surgery should be avoided. Necessary medications should therefore be taken in crushed or liquid form. Slow-release medications must not be crushed, and they should be replaced by the equivalent in divided doses of standard pills. Potassium tablets are notably toxic to the esophagus and the narrow gastric pouch. However, because fluid intake is so restricted early after bariatric surgery, the diuretic therapy may be withheld and potassium supplements may therefore be unnecessary. Bariatric patients commonly use NSAIDs because obesity markedly contributes to degenerative joint disease. In addition, antiinflammatory medications are particularly effective in obesity possibly because it is a proinflammatory state. Liquid ibuprofen avoids the problem of a large pill becoming lodged in the esophagus or gastric pouch, but it does not avoid the systemic effect of NSAIDs on gastric mucosa.

The need for antihypertensives frequently diminishes abruptly after surgery. Most patients may safely discontinue them for a few weeks. In approximately 50% of cases, hypertension is abolished for a long term, but there is a tendency for blood pressure to rise some years afterward despite early normalization as weight is lost. Blood glucose level tends to be reduced rapidly after surgery, and almost 80% of patients will have long-term remission of type 2 diabetes mellitus.[6] In the immediate postoperative period, caloric intake is so low that hypoglycemia might be precipitated by regular doses of medications. Patients taking insulin are usually discharged on half their preoperative dose, with instructions about how to adjust the dose relative to the fasting and postprandial blood glucose levels. Early follow-up with an internist or endocrinologist is arranged.

Weight loss after gastric bypass is rapid in the first few weeks, often averaging 0.5 kg per day in the beginning. After adjustable gastric banding, the weight loss is typically much slower. Adjustments to the gastric band begin about 6 weeks after surgery and every 3 to 8 weeks thereafter until the correct degree of restriction is achieved. The ideal status is when the patient is conscious of a slight degree of restriction but can eat a wide range of foods while being satisfied with smaller quantities. Adjustments are performed by injecting the subcutaneous port with saline using a Huber-type needle. The adjustments are often performed in the surgeon's office, but some programs recommend fluoroscopically guided band adjustments.

Laboratory studies may be ordered after the first 2 to –3 months to follow up the patient's nutritional status. A typical panel should include a complete blood count to check for hemoglobin (Hb) level and mean corpuscular volume (MCV); a comprehensive metabolic panel should include the level of albumin and liver enzymes, level of iron and total iron binding capacity, and levels of vitamin B_{12}, folate, calcium, intact parathyroid hormone (PTH), and 25-hydroxy vitamin D (25-OH vitamin D). A lipid panel is added if the patient had dyslipidemia preoperatively, and HbA1c levels are measured in patients with diabetes. These parameters should be followed up sequentially over several years, as individual abnormalities may be insignificant but a worsening trend implies the need for corrective action.

MEDIUM-TERM FOLLOW-UP

Progress over the next 2 years becomes harder to maintain as patients cease to attend regular office visits. Most bariatric programs struggle to maintain follow-up beyond 2 years, even though follow-up up to 5 years is recommended by the ASMBS to grant Center of Excellence status.[7] Very few publications report on follow-up longer than 2 years after surgery.[8] Follow-up is expensive and may not be reimbursed by the patient's insurance. Patients may have come from a long distance to have surgery in a center of excellence, and they may find it too inconvenient to travel frequently to a large referral center, particularly when they are not experiencing any problems. After substantial weight loss, patients frequently change jobs, or become employed, or undergo other major social and family changes and move away from the area.

The focus of follow-up after the initial period of healing is threefold: monitoring weight loss, assessing resolution of comorbidities, and checking for unwanted effects of the surgery, symptomatic and asymptomatic. Major organizations such as ASMBS recommend visits at 3, 6, and 12 months and annually thereafter, but this is the minimal requirement for patients who are not reporting problems, and in practice most bariatric programs schedule visits more frequently. Lastly, this midterm period is usually the optimal time to refer the patient for plastic surgery to excise redundant skin folds in the anterior abdominal wall, upper arms, medial thighs, and breasts.[9]

Weight Loss

Weight generally stabilizes by 12 to 15 months in patients with lesser degrees of obesity (BMI<50 at the time of surgery) but may take 2 years to level out in superobese patients. Weight loss is most often expressed as percentage of excess weight lost, and the nadir often occurs in the second postoperative year, when up to 75% of excess weight is often lost.[10,11] Thereafter, a small increase in weight occurs, but ideally it should remain stable. After LAGB, the weight loss is slower, and the nadir less profound than after RYGB, and figures around 50% excess body weight loss are commonly reported. Weight loss does appear to be improved by such factors as attendance at support groups and other motivational forums, such as structured physical activity with a trainer or exercise physiologist. Physicians should be aware of the need for continued psychosocial support to help patients maximize the benefits of the surgery. The first year after bariatric surgery can be conceptualized as a "honeymoon" period during which new lifestyle changes can be introduced, which are easier to maintain because they are occurring in the context of success. This is in marked contrast to their experience before surgery, when such attempts met with failure and thus were not maintained.

Resolution of Comorbidities

In broad terms, resolution of comorbidities parallels weight loss, but some metabolic abnormalities such as type 2 diabetes mellitus improve long before much weight has been lost. However, improvement in mobility and degenerative joint disease, sleep apnea, and urinary continence is dependent on actual weight loss.[12] Surgeons rarely manage these conditions, but many programs develop a network of specialist physicians who care for these problems and who have good communication with the bariatric surgeon's office. The major comorbid diseases of interest to the gastroenterologist are gastroesophageal reflux disease (GERD) and nonalcoholic fatty liver disease (NAFLD). GERD is usually totally resolved by contemporary RYGB, because the tiny gastric pouch has minimal acid secretion, which occurs most likely because the antrum has been bypassed and food-stimulated gastrin secretion does not occur.[13] The relief from GERD is usually so marked after RYGB that the recurrence of genuine GERD symptoms should prompt the physician to search for a gastrogastric fistula.

LAGB frequently improves GERD symptoms, but if the band is placed too low or slips distally allowing a pouch of stomach above it to be partially obstructed, GERD may actually be exacerbated. The DS operation also has the potential to exacerbate reflux, especially if overzealous resection of the stomach near the gastroesophageal junction impairs function of the lower esophageal sphincter (**Fig. 2**).

NAFLD is almost always present in severely obese patients, and several studies have shown improvement in liver histology and resolution of many of the pathologic features after serious weight loss. Older discredited operations, such as the jejunoileal bypass, actually worsened liver pathology and sometimes led to cirrhosis, but this has become largely irrelevant to contemporary practice because there are few remaining patients with this outmoded reconstruction. There are a few anecdotal reports of liver cirrhosis developing after the DS, but the incidence seems to be extremely low. Typical laboratory studies always include liver function tests, and minor degrees of transaminitis generally resolve.[14]

Unwanted effects developing or persisting during this time are either related to GI dysfunction or some form of nutritional loss. A few patients continue to report nausea and vomiting over a prolonged period. This nausea and vomiting should not be assumed to be a result of persistence of old eating habits but should prompt a search for a mechanical cause. Strictures of the anastomosis continue to occur even years afterward, for reasons similar to those mentioned earlier, and are usually easy to dilate. If a narrow scope cannot be negotiated past the stricture, a gentle dilation with a 12- to

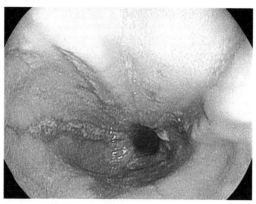

Fig. 2. Severe esophagitis 5 years after DS.

14-mm balloon generally allows safe passage of the scope distally. A somewhat larger balloon can then be positioned accurately across the stricture without fear of more distal perforation. Once the stricture is dilated sufficiently to visualize the entire anastomosis, further dilation up to 20 mm can be undertaken unless there is a large ulcer. Such patients are more safely managed by graduated dilations for a few weeks.

In a few patients, persistent abdominal pain is troublesome. It may be due to intermittent self-limiting bowel obstruction or the postoperative development of gallstones. Both of these causes generally produce episodic pain rather than continuous pain. Abdominal CT scans are helpful in detecting small bowel dilation, but it is important to inform the radiologist of the patient's surgical reconstruction. Gallstones are generally simple to detect on ultrasound, and the surgical solution is also simple. It is difficult and sometimes impossible to do endoscopic retrograde cholangiopancreatography after RYGB, so intraoperative cholangiography is frequently recommended at the time of cholecystectomy.

The occasional patient with persistent unremitting abdominal pain is a challenge for every surgeon and physician. The underlying addictive personality of some bariatric patients can lead to a situation in which there is pressure to provide escalating doses of narcotic pain medication, and this is usually an unhappy situation for all parties.

Complications specific to LAGB include erosion and slippage. Erosion occurs when the band gradually erodes into the stomach lumen. The most frequent mode of presentation is tracking of infection distally toward the port site. Pain, redness, or discharge from the port site should not be assumed to be a result of local infection, and it should prompt endoscopic evaluation, when a characteristically discolored portion of Silastic will be seen just below the gastroesophageal junction. Slippage presents with chest pain, dysphagia, and vomiting. If such a patient presents to an internist or gastroenterologist, it is best to send the patient to the operating surgeon, who will generally deflate the band. If removal of all fluid from the port does not bring about relief, surgical removal or revision is usually required.

Nutritional Complications

Malnutrition, once the "Achilles heel" of bariatric surgery, only rarely complicates contemporary operations. Restriction and malabsorption can contribute to malnutrition, but in patients who remain in follow-up programs, the restrictive element is rarely a significant problem over the long term. The dangers are maximal early in the postoperative period when the patient may experience repetitive vomiting and become thiamine deficient. In the long term, vitamin B_{12} deficiency is a major risk of RYGB because the production of intrinsic factor by the small gastric pouch is so reduced. Supplementation by regular monthly or bimonthly injections or daily sublingual B_{12} tablets is easy, and neurologic impairment from B_{12} deficiency should not occur. Routine examination in the clinic may include testing for vibration sense with a large tuning fork, to check for posterior column loss.

In contrast, malabsorptive operations such as BPD and DS lead to protein-calorie malnutrition in up to 5% of cases, often developing several years after surgery.[15] Such patients typically present with a triad of excessive weight loss, hypoalbuminemic edema, and diarrhea. Despite these severe symptoms, the patients are so terrified of regaining weight that they often resist dietary measures to improve their caloric intake and are reluctant to consider any form of surgical revision. In practice, partial reversal of the BPD or DS is a simple operation in which the alimentary (Roux) limb and the biliopancreatic limb are simply anastomosed more proximally. It occasionally leads to marked weight gain, but in most cases it is about 7 kg.

Calcium metabolism

Difficulty in absorbing calcium and iron is common to all bypass operations, whether RYGB or DS. A strongly positive Chvostek sign not present preoperatively may indicate severe hypocalcemia, which is further studied by measuring PTH and 25-OH vitamin D. The serum calcium and albumin levels are routinely measured in the typical comprehensive metabolic panel. Even in an asymptomatic patient, it is wise to check these levels regularly because the symptoms may develop only gradually although bone loss is inexorably occurring. It is hard to maintain normal vitamin D levels by oral ingestion of supplements; most vitamin D is synthesized by the action of sunlight on the skin, and patients should be encouraged to have regular solar exposure for a few minutes every day. It is now recognized that vitamin D levels should optimally be greater than 30 ng/mL, and vitamin D is frequently subnormal even before surgery. Severe vitamin D deficiency is characterized by proximal muscle weakness in addition to other signs of calcium deficiency and is frequently misattributed to entities such as fibromyalgia. Because vitamin D is a fat-soluble vitamin, its absorption is more problematic after malabsorptive operations such as DS than after RYGB.

Iron, B12, and folate

Anemia is common after all forms of bariatric surgery, but particularly after any kind of bypass. The normal site of iron absorption (duodenum and proximal jejunum) is excluded from the food stream, and the facilitating effect of gastric acid is also lost. Further, the largest subgroup of patients undergoing bariatric surgery is premenopausal women, who are already at risk from iron-deficiency anemia. Consequently, regular iron supplements should be prescribed and the response followed up. The typical pattern on testing is microcytic anemia (MCV<70 fL). The most widely available form of iron supplement is ferrous sulfate, but it is also the form that is most likely to produce abdominal discomfort and constipation. Ferrous gluconate is often easier to tolerate. Typical doses are 50 to 60 mg twice daily. Patients who are compliant with medications and who remain anemic are usually referred to a hematologist for parenteral iron infusions.[16] It is important to inquire about menstrual losses and refer to the patient to a gynecologist if excessive bleeding is present, because endometrial ablation or even hysterectomy may be appropriate.

Folate deficiency is rare in compliant patients because it is easily absorbed. Absorption of B_{12} is poor after RYGB, as described earlier, but is rarely a problem after DS or

LAGB. All bariatric patients should be encouraged to take a daily multivitamin, and supplemental B_{12}, iron, and calcium are advocated if indicated by laboratory studies.

Summary of Management of the Patient with Suspected Malnutrition

If a review of the clinical and laboratory test values indicates malnutrition, the priority is to ensure compliance with follow-up and adequate supplementation. The next step is to correct excessive restriction; patients who report frequent vomiting or regurgitation of foam should be offered endoscopy with dilation. After compliance and restriction are adequately dealt with, the surgeon should consider reducing the degree of malabsorption.

LONG-TERM FOLLOW-UP

After 2 years, it is assumed that the most serious problems would have already manifested, and patients and physicians alike tend to become complacent about follow-up care. Three major elements in long-term care nevertheless require attention: (1) the development of progressive nutritional deficiencies, (2) weight regain and recurrence of comorbidities, and (3) recognition of rare or sporadic complications.

Progressive Development of Nutritional Deficiencies

Deficiency of any of the nutrients mentioned earlier in the article may pose problems years after surgery, especially in patients who no longer attend regular follow-up. When the surgeon no longer has regular contact with the patient, primary care physicians and other internists may be given the responsibility. The annual physician's visit for such patients must include measurement of the laboratory studies outlined earlier. Bone density tests are now a routine part of primary care, and if there is evidence of bone loss, nutritional supervision should be intensified.

Weight Regain

Weight regain is emerging as the greatest threat in the long-term management of bariatric surgery. There is no clear consensus on the exact incidence or severity, but it is estimated that more than 20% of patients will regain a large proportion of the weight initially lost and reenter the category of morbid obesity.[17] Why some patients regain weight is not known, but the 2 broad categories of reasons are (1) surgical factors and (2) lifestyle factors. The major surgical factors are the size of the pouch and the size of the anastomosis. When both are small, as they are generally made these days, the regain of weight is reduced. Large pouches and wider anastomoses allow greater food intake with less satiety. Sometimes the pouch is larger than the size that the surgeon intended it to be because a hiatal hernia was not recognized at the time of surgery.

It is widely believed, largely on anecdotal evidence, that behavioral factors are the most important factors in weight regain. Patients who do not use the honeymoon period to bring about major changes in eating and exercise patterns will gain weight in subsequent years when the restriction has worn off. Sometimes the inability to eat leads to the development of other addictions such as alcohol. Other stressful social factors, such as divorce or loss of employment, may push patients in the direction of their old habits.

The treatment of weight regain is problematic for several reasons. There may be no clear anatomic explanation. Operative revision in such cases may bring about some weight loss initially, but may only set the stage for subsequent recurrent weight gain. Further, most insurance companies deny requests for authorization to perform revisional bariatric surgery for weight regain. Only if a complication such as GERD is found will the company generally authorize it. If there is no clear abnormality to correct, the surgical strategy has been whimsically summarized as "bypassing the band, and banding the bypass."[18] Patients with unsatisfactory weight loss after LAGB may be converted to RYGB, but the risk of leakage is higher. Failure of the RYGB has been reported to respond to placement of a laparoscopic band round the gastric pouch to reimpose a sense of restriction. However, both these strategies are only reported in case series with limited follow-up and so are recommended only on an individualized basis.

In concert with weight regain is the recent recognition that type 2 diabetes sometimes recurs. Even when it does, it is rarely as severe as it was preoperatively. The incidence is not known, but it may be as high as 30% of patients who had diabetes and who experienced relief early after surgery.

Sporadic Complications

Small bowel obstruction can occur at any time after any abdominal surgery but is especially well known after bypass surgery. Adhesions causing a partial volvulus of small bowel, or herniation of bowel into a mesenteric space behind the biliopancreatic limb, are the most likely sources. A unique form of small bowel obstruction may affect patients with the DS, when the biliopancreatic limb becomes obstructed (**Fig. 3**). This obstruction presents with severe central abdominal pain, although normal bowel movements may be preserved; it may progress rapidly to intestinal ischemia and gangrene if not decompressed because it is a closed-loop obstruction. Because this obstruction is not accessible to nasogastric suction or endoscopic decompression, it requires urgent surgery. Consequently, a patient presenting with severe abdominal pain after DS should have an immediate CT scan of the abdomen to check for dilated loops of the biliopancreatic limb.

Hypoglycemia associated with excessive insulin secretion has been reported after RYGB and has been attributed to nesidioblastosis, possibly mediated by the effect of glucagon-like peptide 1 on the pancreas.[19] It presents with episodes of altered mental status associated with profound hypoglycemia and seems to occur in those who were nondiabetic at first. Any patient reporting symptoms suggestive of episodic hypoglycemia should be provided with a home glucose monitor and instructed on its use over a period of several days, to document if hypoglycemia is actually occurring. This simple step often eliminates hypoglycemia as a diagnosis. The workup for

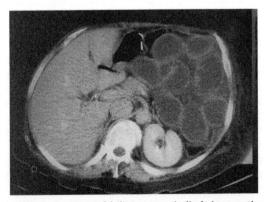

Fig. 3. CT scan showing obstruction of biliopancreatic limb in a patient with a DS. Note multiple fluid-filled loops without contrast.

hypoglycemia is complex, and because the episodes can have serious consequences, prompt referral to an endocrinologist is recommended.

SUMMARY

It is unrealistic for surgeons to follow up all their patients for the rest of their lives. Nevertheless, a long-term ongoing follow-up is critical if the benefits of bariatric surgery are to be sustained and not offset by complications related to the surgery. All involved in the care of these patients must establish a close dialog and provide standard long-term ongoing assessments.

REFERENCES

1. Buchwald HJ, Williams SJ. Bariatric surgery worldwide 2003. Obes Surg 2003;14: 1157–64.
2. Podnos YD, Jimenez JC, Wilson SE, et al. Complications after laparoscopic gastric bypass: a review of 3464 cases. Arch Surg 2003;138:957–61.
3. Derzie AJ, Silvestri F, Liriano E, et al. Wound closure technique and acute wound complications in gastric surgery for morbid obesity: a prospective randomized trial. J Am Coll Surg 2000;191:238–43.
4. Aasheim ET. Wernicke encephalopathy after bariatric surgery: a systematic review. Ann Surg 2004;248:714–20.
5. Mitchell MT, Gasparaitis AE, Alverdy JC. Imaging findings in Roux-en-O and other misconstructions: rare but serious complications of Roux-en-Y Gastric Bypass Surgery. Am J Roentgenol 2008;190:367–73.
6. Schauer PR, Burguera B, Ikramuddin S, et al. Effect of laparoscopic Roux-en Y gastric bypass on type 2 diabetes mellitus. Ann Surg 2003;238(4):467–84.
7. Available at: http://www.surgicalreview.org/pcoe/tertiary/tertiary_provisional.aspx. Accessed January 16, 2010.
8. Buchwald H, Avodor Y, Braunwald E, et al. Bariatric surgery. A systematic review and meta-analysis. JAMA 2004;292:1724–37.
9. Gusenoff JA, Rubin JP. Plastic surgery after weight loss: current concepts in massive weight loss surgery. Aesthet Surg J 2008;28(4):452–5.
10. Strain GW, Gagner M, Pomp A, et al. Comparison of weight loss and body composition changes with four surgical procedures. Surg Obes Relat Dis 2009; 5:582–7.
11. Anthone GJ, Lord RV, DeMeester TR, et al. The duodenal switch operation for the treatment of morbid obesity. Ann Surg 2003;238:618–27.
12. Haines K, Nelson L, Gonzales T, et al. Objective evidence that bariatric surgery improves obesity-related obstructive sleep apnea. Surgery 2007;141:354–8.
13. Patterson EJ, Davis DG, Khajanchee Y, et al. Comparison of objective outcomes following laparoscopic Nissen fundoplication versus laparoscopic gastric bypass in the morbidly obese with heartburn. Surg Endosc 2003;17(10):1561–5.
14. Mattar SG, Velcu LM, Rabinovitz M, et al. Surgically-induced weight loss significantly improves nonalcoholic fatty liver disease and the metabolic syndrome. Ann Surg 2005;242:610–20.
15. Hamoui N, Chock B, Anthone GJ, et al. Revision of the duodenal switch: technique, indications, and outcome. J Am Coll Surg 2007;204(4):603–8.
16. Varma S, Baz W, Badine E, et al. Need for parenteral iron therapy after bariatric surgery. Surg Obes Relat Dis 2008;4(6):715–9.
17. Meguid M, Glade M, Middleton F. Weight regain after Roux-en-Y: a significant 20% complication related to PYY. Nutrition 2008;24:832–42.

18. Carpenter RO, Williams DB, Richards WO. Laparoscopic adjustable gastric banding after previous Roux-en-Y gastric bypass. Surg Obes Relat Dis 2009. [Epub ahead of print].
19. Service GJ, Thompson GB, Service FJ, et al. Hyperinsulinemic hypoglycemia with nesidioblastosis after gastric-bypass surgery. N Engl J Med 2005;353: 249–54.

Index

Note: Page numbers of article titles are in **boldface** type.

A

Abdominal obesity
  esophageal disorders in, 30
  measurement of, 2
Abdominal pain
  after bariatric surgery, 92, 141
  in obesity, 9–22
Adenocarcinoma, esophageal, 30, 41–42
Adenomatous polyps, of colon, 31, 52–52
Agouti-related peptides, in appetite regulation, 27
Androgens, colorectal neoplasia and, 49
Anemia, after bariatric surgery, 118–121, 142–143
Anorexiants, mechanism of action of, 28
Antireflux surgery, for GERD, 43
Appetite, regulation of, 24–28
Arcuate nucleus, in appetite regulation, 27

B

Bacterial overgrowth, after bariatric surgery, 29, 122
Band migration, after bariatric surgery, 93
Bariatric surgery
  comorbid condition management after, 138–141
  complications of, 92–94, 125–133
    gastrointestinal dysfunction, 28–29, 137–138
    incisional problems, 136–137
    metabolic, 109–113
    nutritional, 109–111, 113–122, 141–143
    sporadic, 144–145
    weight regain, 94, 143–144
  endoscopy after, 89–94
  ERCP after, **99–107**
  failure of, 94, 143–144
  follow-up after, **135–146**
    long-term, 143–145
    medium-term, 139–143
    short-term, 136–139
  gut hormone levels after, 29–30
  in fatty liver disease, 61
  preoperative assessment before, **81–86**
  procedures for, 89–92, **125–133**. *See also individual procedures.*

Gastroenterol Clin N Am 39 (2010) 147–156
doi:10.1016/S0889-8553(10)00010-5
0889-8553/10/$ – see front matter © 2010 Elsevier Inc. All rights reserved.

gastro.theclinics.com

Moving?

Make sure your subscription moves with you!

To notify us of your new address, find your **Clinics Account Number** (located on your mailing label above your name), and contact customer service at:

E-mail: elspcs@elsevier.com

800-654-2452 (subscribers in the U.S. & Canada)
314-453-7041 (subscribers outside of the U.S. & Canada)

Fax number: 314-523-5170

Elsevier Periodicals Customer Service
11830 Westline Industrial Drive
St. Louis, MO 63146

*To ensure uninterrupted delivery of your subscription, please notify us at least 4 weeks in advance of move.

Printed and bound by CPI Group (UK) Ltd, Croydon, CR0 4YY

03/10/2024

01040447-0015